The Val...
Everything

Social Work and i... Importance
in the Field of ...ental Health

Peter Gilbert

RHP

Russell House Publishing

First published in 2003 by:
Russell House Publishing Ltd.
4 St George's House
Uplyme Road
Lyme Regis
Dorset DT7 3LS

Tel: 01297-443948
Fax: 01297-442722
e-mail: help@russellhouse.co.uk
www.russellhouse.co.uk

© Peter Gilbert

British Library Cataloguing-in-publication Data:
A catalogue record for this book is available from the British Library.

ISBN: 1-903855-24-1

Typeset by TW Typesetting, Plymouth, Devon

Printed by Cromwell Press, Trowbridge

Russell House Publishing
is a group of social work, probation, education and youth and community work practitioners and academics working in collaboration with a professional publishing team.
Our aim is to work closely with the field to produce innovative and valuable materials to help managers, trainers, practitioners and students.
We are keen to receive feedback on publications and new ideas for future projects.
For details of our other publications please visit our website or ask us for a catalogue. Contact details are on this page.

Contents

To
Sue, Mary, Joanna and Ruth

Foreword

Social care, and more narrowly social work, is not a straightforward field to communicate to the uninitiated. In the mass media, it is all-too-often associated with either dangerous incompetence or over-zealous political correctness. Social workers themselves are frequently denigrated by newspapers when they fail, yet completely invisible when they succeed.

Unlike nurses, doctors and teachers, social workers are rarely recognised for their professionalism and dedication to the public good. Whereas using the NHS is something we are mostly happy to do, being in contact with social services is seen by many as a sign of failure, of exclusion. There is thus little incentive to speak up for a profession that works with society's most marginalised, isolated and vulnerable members.

For these reasons, the value of social work is too often hidden from the public view. This book sets the record straight. It provides a fascinating case for the vital role played by social workers in the treatment, care and support of people with mental health needs.

At the core is the imperative for social work practitioners to see the person with whom they work as a whole human being within a complex society. Where some other professions may be encouraged to see only a part of the person, everything in a social worker's training and experience causes them to look at the bigger picture and to respond to needs not met by other services.

Such a role also means that social work is uniquely exposed to changing opinions and actions. For example, yesterday's taboos are today's accepted lifestyles, but some new opportunities pose new challenges and certain types of behaviour are no longer tolerated. Consider the access the internet allows and its consequences, and the ever growing intolerance of risk in any manifestation.

This book gives clear illustration of the changing expectations of social work. It shows also powerfully that the role and status of social work are determined by wider social, political and economic forces. More than any other profession I can think of, the boundaries of social work are not fixed in stone but a result of historical change – influenced by shifts in political priorities, social needs, economic constraints and academic learning. Those shifts continue today.

Social services now face an uncertain future. The impact of forthcoming changes to mental health law and the structures under which social care is delivered could be far-reaching. This is why the lack of public and political respect and understanding for social work is so crucial. However, one point we can be very certain about. The need for social care will not disappear, and even if we rename or restructure, many of the interventions and services will remain crucial to the survival of the most vulnerable in society.

Finally, I hope that this wonderful book, loaded with great anecdotes and personal experiences, will not only engage its readers, but also achieve a moment of reflection why we are all committed to caring.

Dr Matt Muijen, Chief Executive,
Sainsbury Centre for Mental Health

Introduction

This is an unprecedented time for mental health as a declared national priority, with well-developed and progressive policies and targeted resources. Increasingly, mental health is seen as a crucial issue for a healthy and productive nation; the mental as well as physical health of citizens is seen as a vital component in the regeneration of communities; and campaigns are in place to create a more positive image of and focus on mental well-being, mental illness and recovery. It has been interesting over the last year to see the popularity of films such as *Iris* and *A Beautiful Mind* tackling the demanding issues of dementia and schizophrenia respectively.

Progress, however, is set against a background of historical cul-de-sacs in terms of policy and service development; regular moral panics; past under-investment pessimism and a workforce under considerable strain at a time when the demographic tide is running away from us.

Investment in new programmes and additional staff are coming into place at a time of major structural upheaval in the organisations – both health and social care – which deliver services to individuals, families and communities. A challenge facing any kind of organisation is how to retain and motivate a scarce number of skilled staff and encapsulate values and skills when the structures around them are undergoing major change. Social work is a profession facing this challenge at present, as mental health appears to be moving more towards the NHS in terms of its organisational home; the value of social work generally has been challenged, and central and local government have had to produce a specific campaign to bring people into the profession; social workers are often a numerically small part of a wider mental health workforce; and the specific role of the 'Approved Social Worker' is under question in the reform of mental health legislation, currently under discussion.

This book considers the value of social work in the light of what users and carers want from services, and the value base of the new policies for reform; the role of the social worker in different settings; and ways of taking these values and skills forward into new settings. I hope that it will provide a boost to the confidence of social workers by reinforcing the tremendous resource they are to people in the greatest need in our society; and also help colleagues in the new mental health trusts and in other statutory and voluntary agencies value the contribution social work can bring.

Peter Gilbert
December 2002

Biographical Note

Peter Gilbert was a social work practitioner in various settings for 13 years, and practised as a duly authorised officer under the 1959 Mental Health Act and as an ASW under the 1983 Act.

Following a first career in the army and a degree in modern history from Balliol College, Oxford, Peter became a trainee social worker with West Sussex County Council and worked in a variety of settings with all client groups. Qualifying with a master's degree in social work from the University of Sussex, Peter practised as a generic worker, but became increasingly interested in issues around mental health and learning disability. In 1981 he took up a new post as Team Leader at the Forest Hospital for people with learning disabilities; the job had a management, practice, policy, resource-building, hospital reprovision and educational role. During this time, Peter qualified and practised as an ASW (including the out-of-hours call service – usually 2 am!).

A dual strategic and operational post with a London borough was followed by a period managing mental health and other specialist services in Kent, where he also completed an MBA at Roffey Park Management Institute/Sussex University. This was a time of considerable expansion of mental health services and their profile in Kent, and joint work with the NHS.

In May 1992, Peter joined Staffordshire County Council, as Director of Operations, with a brief to bring in the reforms under the NHS and Community Care Act in time for April 1993. A great deal of work was undertaken in Staffordshire by Peter and his team around the closure and reprovision of St Matthews and St Edwards Hospitals, with initiatives on user and carer involvement, alternatives to hospital admission and links with primary care.

Formation of common strategies and approaches with users, carers and partner agencies was evident in Peter's work as Director of Social Services for Worcestershire County Council from December 1997 to April 2001. The social work and social care service in Mental Health and the NHS Trust formed an integrated service at this time.

Following retirement from local government, Peter has worked as a member of the core group setting up the National Institute for Mental Health in England; as Senior Adviser in Social Care for the Sainsbury Centre for Mental Health; as an Associate Consultant with the National Development Team; and with the Shaftesbury Society.

Author of and contributor to several books on social history and policy, practice and management, Peter Gilbert is a visiting Research Fellow at the University of Sussex and an Honorary Research Associate at Staffordshire University. He is a member of the editorial board of MCC, has spoken at and chaired a number of national conferences; and also works with the Worth Abbey Centre for Spirituality, co-running workshops on spirituality and leadership in the workplace. At the beginning of 2002, he co-authored a training pack on supervision and leadership with Professor Neil Thompson.

Currently a member of the new Social Perspectives Network, hosted by TOPSS, Peter has been a member of specialist panels for the English National Board and CCETSW, and from February, 2003 in NIMHE/SCIE Fellow in Social Care (Policy and Practice).

Acknowledgements

One of the profound aspects of Social Work is the creation of valued connections in achieving our goals, so I have a great many people to thank, not just those who have been so generous with their help to me in writing the book but those who have nurtured my educational practice in social work and management, and people who supported me when I experienced an episode of stress and depression in 2000/2001.

Firstly, I would like to thank Dr Matt Muijen, Chief Executive, and Dr Andrew McCulloch, formerly Director of Policy, for the Sainsbury Centre for Mental Health, for recognising the need to address the concerns around social care and social work and commissioning me to write this book. My thanks to both of them for their support during the whole process.

I have been privileged since September 2001 to be working with Professor Anthony Sheehan, Ingrid Steele and James Filton and the core group setting up the National Institute for Mental Health in England. It is always stimulating to be in at the creation of a new project and it has been a very energising and educational experience.

I was very fortunate to have as my first manager in social work, Bridget Ogden, one of the first childcare officers, following from the Curtis Committee and the 1948 Act. Bridget was an outstanding leader with the highest professional integrity and standards, and a major formative influence. The late Jean Carruthers was a superb exemplar as a team manager, as was Colin Brunt and Bob Phipps and Ian Gates as practitioners. I have kept contact with Hugh England, my tutor on the Masters in Social Work course at Sussex University, and whose book *Social Work as Art* has been an ongoing influence on me; and Carol Kedward, also at Sussex University, both of whom have been a continuing inspiration. Professor Neil Thompson has been an ongoing source of advice during the writing of this book, and I am indebted to his admirably clear thinking about Social Work as a profession.

Extended families can be vital to an individual's sound mental health, and I have been fortunate to have the extended family of the monastic and lay communities of the Benedictine Abbey at Worth in Sussex. My special thanks to Dom Luke Jolly, Director of the Centre for Spirituality, Dom Stephen Ortiger, third Abbot of Worth, and his successor, Dom Christopher Jamison.

David Joannides, Director of Social Services for Dorset County Council and chair of the ADSS Mental Health Strategy Group, has been a champion for social work and social care in a changing context, and someone who is always personally supportive and a great sounding board for ideas. My thanks to him and colleagues on the Mental Health Strategy Group, especially Jenny Goodhall, Ted Unsworth, Alan Chittenden and Tim Watts.

I would like to record my debt to all the users and carers I have worked with in twenty-six years in social services, and the way that they have shaped my practice. My special thanks to Simon Henge, Chair of Worcestershire Association of Service Users and his colleagues, and Howard Brooksbank, Chair of Worcestershire Association of Carers and colleagues.

Readers will have noted the historical bent and I would like to acknowledge my debt to the stimulating and challenging teaching of Maurice Keen, Dr Christopher

Hill and Dr Colin Lucas of Balliol College, Oxford, and my first history teacher, Dom Bernard Moss.

Many people, by no means all from a social work and social care background, have been enormously generous with their time and thought. I would like to take the opportunity to thank Jane Campbell (Chairperson), Dr Ray Jones (former Chief Executive), Trish Kearney and Don Brand of the Social Care Institute for Excellence; Margaret Clayton, Chairperson of the Mental Health Act Commission; Bob Lake, Colin Farnworth, Peter Edgerton, Ian Lovatt, Gilly Gilmore, Bill Pierpoint, Trevor Edwards and Alan Lotinga, Bernard Bester and many other colleagues from Staffordshire Social Services; Keith Murray (Director) and Jeremy Pritlove from Leeds Social Services; Sue Hunt (Chief Executive), Jenny Jaynes and Alan Craig, Worcestershire Mental Health Partnership Trust; Ian Dyer, States of Jersey Mental Health Services; Carolyn Merry, Hari Sewell and Kath Tempest, Social Services Inspectorate; Philip Douglas, Joan Elliott and social workers in Northamptonshire; Richard Brook, Chief executive, MIND; Dr Ian McPherson, Director of the West Midlands Development Centre; Melanie Walker and Julie Barton from the St George's and South London Mental Health Trust; Jennifer Barnard (Chair) and Joan Maughan (Chief Executive), the National Development Team; Chief Constable Peter Neyroud, Thames Valley Police; Chief Superintendent Dermot McCann, West Mercia Police; Dr David Shiers, Advisor to NIMHE on Primary Care; John Taylor, NCSC; Bill Robinson , formerly Head of Worcestershire and Herefordshire YOT; Richard Humphries, DoH; George O'Neil, Devon SSD; Julie French, Worcestershire SSD; Mark Viner, Kent County Council; Terry Philpott and Polly Neate, *Community Care*; Austen Ivereigh, *The Tablet*; Phil Gray, Chief Executive the Chartered Society of Physiotherapists; Dr Maggie Keeble, General Practitioner; Chris and Sue Williams; Trish and Terry Haines; Judy Foster from TOPPS, Jerry Tew, Jeannie Molyneaux, Thurstine Bassett, Malcolm Firth, Maria Duggan, Professor Andrew Cooper, Jo Warner and colleagues in the Social Perspectives Network; Roger Mortimore, LGA; Helen Rea and Dr Hugh Middleton from the East Midlands Developments Centre; Bruce Buckley, Director Derby Social Services; the Revd Dr Peter Sedgwick, Board of Social Responsibility; Charles and Fiona Wookey; Sarah Lindsell, Director of CASC; the Right Revd Terry Brain, Bishop of Salford, and other members of the Bishops Social Welfare Committee; Susan Scarth and members of Worcester MIND; Alison Webster and Janice Price from the Diocese of Worcester; Colin Wilson, Northern Centre for Mental Health; Peter Lane, Peterborough Social Services; Dr Ian Cunningham and members of the Self-managed Learning Network; Dr Lynne Friedli, Chief Executive of Mentality; Dr Karen Linde, Leeds University; Suki Desai, University of Wolverhampton; Gary Miles, Roffey Park Management Institute; Councillors George Mardle, John Taylor and Peter Pinfield, for their example of combining political skills with integrity in steering through the rapids and shoals of life in Local Government; Jill Manthorpe, Hull University; Bob Hudson from the Nuffield Institute; Chris Parker and Peter Thistlethwaite, *Pavilion Publishing*; Judith Westcott, Jill Garner, Ken Tucker, Liz Lee and the late lamented Neil Walker from the Shaftesbury Society; John Nurse, Sutton Advocacy; Sheila Hollins, Professor of the Psychiatry of Disability, St George's Hospital Medical School; Jo Williams, Director of Social Services, Cheshire County Council; Christina Pond, the NHS Leadership Centre; Rachel Hetherington, Brunel University; Terry Scragg, Southampton University; Dinah Morley and Gavin Baylis from Young Minds;

Michelle Rowett, Chief Executive of the Manic Depression Fellowship; Cliff Prior, Chief Executive of Rethink; the Board of Jersey Focus on Mental Health; Ian Johnson, Director of BASW; Zofia Butrym and member of the CSWG; Dr Judith Laing, Cardiff Law School; Dr Duncan Double, Critical Psychiatry Network; Andy Nash, London Development Centre, NIMHE.

My thanks to Advocate Julian Clyde-Smith for life-long friendship and inviting me back to work on Mental Health issues on the beautiful island of Jersey where I grew up.

One of my 'strategies for living' is running and I would like to thank Mike Sell for his encouragement and friendship, and Nigel Stinton and all members of Worcester Joggers; plus Ken Brooks, Martin Newhill and Stuart Wilde for assisting me in achieving a lifetime ambition in completing the London Marathon at the age of fifty-one!

Lastly, I would like to thank my long-suffering family, and I promise that they can have the dining room back very shortly! My thanks also to Maggie Holloway, who typed the manuscript and who views my handwriting as marginally less decipherable than the average Egyptian hieroglyph!

Chapter 1

Mental Health – Everybody's Issue

Sharing a common humanity

Humour is often a way of cutting to the core of major issues. At a time when the profile of mental health was being raised in the 1950s, the famous pre-satirical duo of Michael Flanders and Donald Swann were a major West End hit with their show 'At the Drop of a Hat'. Flanders, himself disabled by polio, raised the issue of mental ill-health and quipped:

> *Two out of every three people suffer from a mental illness – Luckily there are only two of us!*

Mental illness has had such a stigma attached to it throughout history that most people still find it difficult to admit to any mental distress, and yet the World Health Organisation report, *New Understanding, New Hope* (October 2001), states clearly that one in four people around the world are suffering from a recognised psychiatric illness or behavioural or personality problem at any one time. Depression is likely to become the most prevalent condition in the world over the next ten years. The Director General of the WHO Gro Harlem-Brundtland directly attacked the stigmatisation of mental illness:

> *Mental illness is not a personal failure. In fact, if there is failure, it is to be found in the way we have responded to people with mental and brain disorders. I hope this report will dispel long-held doubts and dogma and mark the beginning of a new public health era in the field of Mental Health.*
>
> WHO, 2001.

Distancing ourselves is not a viable strategy as we are all vulnerable to mental distress of some kind or another, through the inevitable life and traumatic crises that we face as human beings. In a world that is changing at an ever-increasing pace, the pressure on all of us is ever present.

More positively, the 'Mind Out for Mental Health' campaign has begun to acknowledge mental distress as a part of everyday life; the experience as life-changing in a positive as well as a negative way; and the importance of paying attention to our emotional and spiritual well-being. Personal testimonies such as Linda Hart's *Phone at Nine to Say You're Alive* (Hart, 1995) of her experiences of hospitalisation and recovery are particularly helpful as Hart was a

mental health professional and faced the double challenge of being treated by colleagues.

Incidence of mental illness and mental distress

- One in four people will experience some kind of mental health problem during a year.
- 10 to 25 per cent of the general population seek advice from their GP.
- 2 to 4 per cent of the above will have a severe mental illness, while a smaller number will experience severe and enduring mental illness.
- Estimates for the latter vary from 0.3 to 1.5 per cent of the population.
- One in ten children has a recognised mental disorder.
- 90 per cent of young offenders and people in prison have mental health needs.

Neuroses

About ten to 30 per cent of the population suffer from anxiety or depression. It is common to talk very loosely about 'being depressed' these days, but a lowness of mood, stemming from personality type, the organic make-up of the individual, or life pressures or traumas or major changes, can lead on to a clinical condition:

- More than one in ten people are likely to have an anxiety disorder which severely affects their everyday lives, at some stage during their life.
- 13 per cent of the adult population are calculated to experience a phobia, while around 2.5 per cent are likely to have an obsessive compulsive disorder.
- One in ten people are likely to have some form of depression at any one time, while one in 20 people will have a serious or 'clinical depression'.

Psychoses

Recent Department of Health statistics show an incidence of five to six per 1000, but the number of men from the Afro-Caribbean community who were diagnosed as having a psychosis, is much higher. Likewise, the disproportionate use

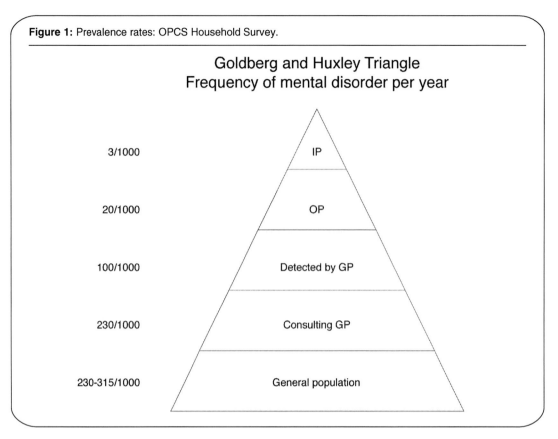

Figure 1: Prevalence rates: OPCS Household Survey.

Goldberg and Huxley Triangle
Frequency of mental disorder per year

3/1000 — IP

20/1000 — OP

100/1000 — Detected by GP

230/1000 — Consulting GP

230-315/1000 — General population

of compulsory orders in relation to young Afro-Caribbean men has been recorded (Cope, 1989).

Schizophrenia

Estimates vary from one to four per cent of the population who may experience schizophrenia.

There is a good chance of people making a good recovery with some form of treatment; two thirds may experience repeat episodes with a need for some support from specialist agencies in between; and ten to 15 per cent will have a severe and enduring mental illness.

Manic depression or bi-polar mood disorder

Approximately one in a 100 adults will experience manic depression. 20 per cent of people who have a first episode do not have another one.

Personality disorder

Fifty-four men per 1000 and 34 women per 1000 have a personality disorder (of whom a very small percentage may have dangerous behaviours).

Substance misuse

Hazardous drinking (25 per cent) and illicit drug use (5–15 per cent) are major causes and complications in mental disorder.

Gender differences

Research demonstrates considerable gender differences, but some of these variances may stem as much from presentation and diagnosis as the reality of the illness:

- 18 per cent of women were found to have had a 'neurotic disorder' such as anxiety, depression, phobias and panic attacks, compared with 11 per cent of men (Office for National Statistics, 1995). The gender differences are less apparent in the later stages of middle age, and are reversed in people aged over 55 years.
- Men are three times more likely to have a dependence on alcohol, and twice as likely to be dependent upon drugs.

- Women are more likely to consult their GP while experiencing anxiety, depression or phobias.
- Men tend to experience psychotic illnesses at an earlier stage in their lives. The response to treatment is often poorer, and the incidence of people with severe and enduring mental illness, following a psychotic breakdown, is much higher among men.

Black and ethnic minorities

> **Case Example 1**
>
> 'Hadley' is a young Afro-Caribbean man who suffered his first psychotic episode while a student at university, and was compulsorily admitted to hospital. His mother, sister and extended family have been very supportive of 'Hadley', but the lack of initial understanding and information about the condition, and concerns about their own safety, meant that by the time of the first hospital admission, relations were extremely strained.
>
> The social worker's involvement came at a time when it looked as though the young man would become increasingly isolated and could become homeless. An appreciation of the social and cultural factors as well as those specific to Hadley's mental illness, meant that the worker was able to increase the tolerance within the family of Hadley's behaviour, help him feel less isolated and stigmatised – the problem had primarily arisen initially due to discrimination he had experienced as a young, black, male, mentally ill student – and secure him appropriate accommodation following good collaboration with housing and welfare rights agencies.
>
> Intensive work, good networking skills, and an ability to understand the complexities of the cultural context, meant that family relationships were repaired and renewed, and that when Hadley experienced periodic recurrences of his illness, services were able to intervene quickly, and in a way acceptable to the user himself.

One of the major issues in this area is that of cultural perception (see Fernando, 1995).

Afro-Caribbeans are twice as likely as Caucasians to be diagnosed with a mental illness, and are three to five times more likely to be diagnosed and admitted to hospital for schizophrenia.

> *The reality is I see myself as 'normal' but a lot of people don't see me as normal. I see other people who have similar experiences as me but they are not seen as mentally ill ... I often question if it's my culture, gender and/or age that gets a negative reaction.*
>
> black service user.

Stanley and Manthorpe, in their trawl through the mental health enquiry reports, comment that in the case of Christopher Clunis, there was 'a tendency for professionals to resort too readily to the stereotype of the young, black man as a drug abuser in their assessments of him' (see Stanley and Manthorpe, 2001: Ritchie et al., 1994).

Mental health in children and young people

There is increasing concern around the diagnosis of autism and behavioural disorders in children and young people, and also the rise in depressive illnesses at an earlier age. One study found a large number of girls with serious depression who were not in contact with specialist services.

- 10 per cent of children and young people are estimated to have mental health problems that require professional intervention.

Mental health in older people

Mental distress and mental illness is often not well identified by professionals, as it is assumed that the memory, energy and buoyancy of people will decline as they age.

In fact, the situation is very complicated with many older people making use of the time they have to engage in activities they have always wanted to do, travel etc., while at the same time increased social mobility in personal and geographical terms has meant many more people living alone and a long way away from their extended families, often leading to problems of isolation.

- It is estimated that 15 per cent of people over 65 have depression, with an estimated five per cent having severe depression. There is a correlation between depression in older people and living alone.

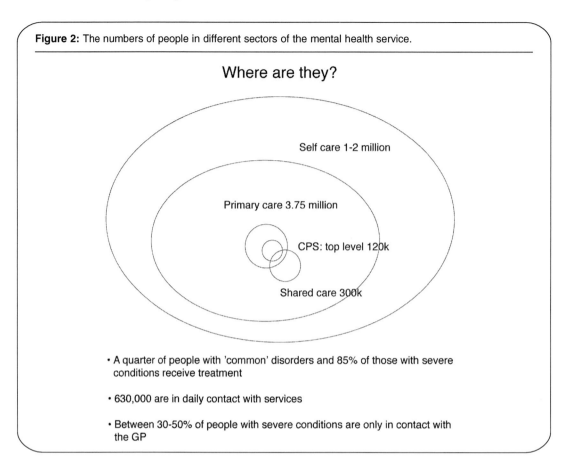

Figure 2: The numbers of people in different sectors of the mental health service.

Where are they?

Self care 1-2 million

Primary care 3.75 million

CPS: top level 120k

Shared care 300k

- A quarter of people with 'common' disorders and 85% of those with severe conditions receive treatment

- 630,000 are in daily contact with services

- Between 30-50% of people with severe conditions are only in contact with the GP

- Dementia affects one per cent of people between 60 and 65 years, 5 per cent of people over 65 and 10 to 20 per cent of people over 80 years old.

Suicide and mental health

Although the reduction of suicides is a target in the National Service Framework, mental ill-health is not a precondition to committing suicide.

Recently, suicide has moved from being the second most common cause of death amongst under 35 year olds to the most prevalent:

- The numbers of male suicides (and deaths that are undetermined but may be suicide) have risen sharply since the late 1970s. Female suicides are falling.
- Despite the caveat above, a high proportion of people who take their own life have a mental illness.
- Living circumstances, childhood experiences, social networks, employment and housing are all major determinants.

Health inequalities

- Depression increases the risk of developing heart disease and having strokes.
- It has an adverse effect on outcomes from asthma, arthritis and diabetes.
- In the case of schizophrenia, standard mortality rate (SMR) is twice the average.

Social and economic inequalities

On the whole, people with a mental health need experience a number of social and economic inequalities, some of which may be cause and others effect:

- A higher proportion are separated or divorced and living alone.
- On average, they have fewer educational qualifications.
- They are less likely to own property.
- Psychoses are more prevalent in the inner cities.

Inequalities in the workplace

- Mental ill-health affects approximately one in five workers.
- Six out of every seven people with a severe mental illness are unable to secure work.
- Those who have been diagnosed as having a mental illness experience greater difficulty in getting insurance, pension cover etc.

The costs to the economy

- £11.8 billion is a cost to the nation in lost employment.
- MIND estimates 91 million working days were lost in 1995.
- The total cost to the economy is over £30 billion pounds.

In the future

People seeking help at times of mental distress and mental disorder are likely to be increasingly more informed, better educated generally and in the specifics around mental health, want quicker access to advice and services and demand greater control and choice in the type of services they are offered. (Information from the Mental Health Foundation, 1999 and the Department of Health).

Incidence of mental distress and mental illness is fundamentally affected by environmental factors such as poverty, crime, employment and community deterioration, housing etc., and cultural factors around ethnicity and belief systems, language, discrimination, segregation, inter-generational and community conflicts.

Social workers have a prime responsibility and the relevant aptitude to ensure that the individual is seen within this wider context so that a full appreciation of their situation and the challenges facing them is gained.

Chapter 2

Society – What Society?!

Margaret Thatcher's well-known, and oft-quoted comment that there is no such thing as society, strikes at the heart of all we know about how individuals, families, neighbourhoods, groups, communities and nations work, and have worked throughout history.

The striking and potent recent photo exhibition: 'One in Four', part of the Department of Health's 'Mind Out for Mental Health' campaign (February 2002) where public figures have 'come out' and spoken about their episodes of mental distress, speaks volumes about them as people, about changing attitudes to mental health, but also the enduring suspicion of and perceived shame of mental ill-health.

> I've suffered from depression all my life . . . The real big one happened about thirty years ago when I suddenly started to lose confidence in my abilities as an actor and as a consequence, gave up the business. Then my daughter was born and it got much, much worse. I had agoraphobia and claustrophobia and couldn't even get out of the door to go shopping . . . There wasn't really anyone there for me at that time. It wasn't so much a lack of sympathy as a lack of understanding . . . After about a year, I remember waking up one morning and thinking 'I can't stand living in this circumscribed way any longer' so I threw the pills down the loo and ran round the block out of frustration and rage. It was the start to getting better and getting back to work.
>
> actress, Stephanie Cole, quoted in
> Mental Health Today, March 2002.

I have recently been undertaking some independent work with voluntary organisations on an island community. Service users made it clear that stigma was a major issue within the restricted population, where it was felt people had access to knowledge about other people's business more readily. Sometimes, small can be 'claustrophobic' as well as 'beautiful'! On the other hand, the island had many advantages. A unique system of government, laws, social institutions, welfare and culture, where policy and legislation can be influenced by a wide range of opinion-formers in an inclusive way, which is much more difficult in a larger nation state.

The size and sense of identity on the island means that its service delivery in all the areas essential to well-being: employment, housing, leisure, social groups, faith communities etc., can be worked upon in such a way that front line service delivery is sensitised to the needs of vulnerable people.

> I quite agree that influencing what they call 'the top people' is the first step to make things work for you, but it's no good if that change of heart doesn't reach down to the people you meet face-to-face.
>
> service user talking about welfare benefits.

It is even more essential that professionals and professional bodies work creatively and harmoniously together. Significantly, the island has brought health and social care together in one agency, with the Community Division clearly determined to encapsulate a social perspective.

Stigma

Societies, their proportions, identity, history, culture and values, clearly influence how the most vulnerable citizens (and whether the society regards particular groups as fellow citizens at all is crucial here) are regarded and related to; and, as Mahatma Ghandi stated 'A civilisation or society must be judged by the care it gives to its weakest and most under-privileged members' (quoted in Gilbert and Scragg, 1992).

The late Roy Porter, the social historian, in his recently published book: *Madness: A Brief History* (Porter, 2002: p62–3) revisits Irving Goffman (Goffman, 1970) who spoke about stigma as the creation of spoiled identity and the disqualification of persons from full social acceptance.

Individuals and groups partake of this stigmatisation because:

- Our insecurities demand we distance ourselves from those who are different from us: health (physical or mental), race, colour, creed, foreign nationals, gay/straight, outsiders etc.
- Placing some into a metaphysical 'ghetto' makes us feel as though we are whole, the 'in crowd', secure, successful etc.

The American novelist, Ursula Le Guin, has a beautifully wry look at these issues in her short story, *S.Q.*, where an American government takes the advice of an influential psychologist and introduces a Sanity Quotient. Very soon, far more people are in the institutional camps for those who have 'failed' the sanity quotient than are outside it! At the end of the novel, the psychologist himself is committed and his personal assistant runs America single-handed! (Le Guin, 1984).

Porter's work demonstrates the effect of societal perceptions and values on how people with a mental illness are responded to, and that a traditional, progressive ('Whiggish') approach to history is far too sanguine. Kathleen Jones, in her seminal work, *A History of the Mental Health Services*, writes that:

> It is important to recognise that the way in which the mentally ill . . . are defined and cared for is primarily a social response to a very basic set of human problems . . . How do we define (mental health)? What forms of care should the community provide? Who should be responsible for administering them? What is liberty, and how can it best be safeguarded? All societies have these problems. How they answer them depends on what they are, and the **values** they hold.
>
> Jones, 1972: pxiii (my emphasis).

Historical trends

History is not a fashionable subject but it is a vital way of identifying patterns, themes and cycles of social activity. In Britain there could be said to be five common strands to the responses to the challenges which human groups face:

- Some balance of public and private provision is normally to be found.
- There are compromises as to whether the services are organised centrally or at a more local level.
- There are constant debates as to whether treatments should be delivered personally, at home for instance, or whether recipients should be treated in institutions.
- Likewise decisions to be made about making provision in cash or kind.
- The liberty of the individual versus their safety and that of the public is a constant issue.

adapted from Midwinter, 1994.

It is well worth keeping these things in mind as public policy in Britain tends to oscillate abruptly between extremes.

Public versus private

The legislation introduced by the Earl of Shaftesbury in the 19th century was partly as a reaction to the abuses of the private madhouses (see Parry-Jones, 1972) but the county asylums moved from being, as Jones wrote 'the system to the System' (Jones, 1972: pxii). The dead hand of an overwhelming public monopoly, with minimal oversight and support, spawned as many problems as it solved.

The current political battles over the mixed economy are in part a reaction to the American-style laissez-faire economics of the 1980s.

Central versus local

Health and social care are prime examples of the tendency to gyrate between control from the centre, with clarity of direction, but loss of local initiative, and local autonomy, which can result in the 'post code lottery' often complained about by public and politicians alike.

When Aneuran Bevan launched the new National Health Service in 1948, he remarked that if a bedpan fell on a hospital floor the noise would resound in the Palace of Westminster (Jenkins, 1996). In March of this year, Alan Milburn, Secretary of State for Health, proclaimed:

> I do not believe a million strong services can be run from Whitehall. Half a century of experience shows us that this approach limits local leadership and stifles local initiative . . . Where our first term in office was concerned with putting a national framework in place, this second term is about introducing new incentives, encouraging greater local innovation and stimulating more patient choice.
>
> speech to the Allied Health professions and Health Care scientists, National Leadership Conference, 13th March 2002.

Local authority social services are much more likely to be framed by local choices, driven by political or interest group decisions. Joint reviews by the Audit Commission/SSI Joint Review Team, often find considerable response to locally expressed need, but the downside is that citizens who move from the city of Seamouth to the market town of Blankton cannot understand why the range and depth of services is so different in the two local authorities.

National Service Frameworks; the infrastructure of new national institutions for regulation and/or quality improvement (especially those developmental agencies with local centres such as in the case of SCIE and NIMHE) and the development of major charitable policy institutes such as SCMH, bring with them a chance that the pendulum will cease to oscillate so violently and a balance between national strategy and local innovation and responsiveness can be accomplished.

Treatment at home or in institutions

It would seem axiomatic to state that the former is now the dominant paradigm. The NHS and Community Care Act of 1990 was meant to see a greater reliance on domiciliary care for vulnerable adults; Quality Protects places great emphasis on family-based care for children; we are meant to be in a 'Primary Care-led NHS'; and the investment in mental health services over the next three years will be in terms of early intervention, assertive outreach and primary care teams.

All the evidence points to a need to support, sustain and improve people's living and social skills in the environments in which they live, but there are always financial and other incentives, and societal pressures, which have led for example to an increase in the number of looked-after children and in some areas a decline in home care, as opposed to the residential solutions, in the care of older people, including those with mental health needs (evidenced by the Audit Commission to the Commons Health Select Committee, reported in the *Health Service Journal*, 28th March 2002).

In Mental Health, much of the investment in the old county asylum/psychiatric hospitals, which as historians have pointed out was a major capital and revenue commitment, were siphoned off into other NHS services or savings, which has left the public often suspicious of community-based solutions. 'Care in the Community' became a term to denote neglect rather than care in all the TV soaps during the 1990s. But when the then Secretary of State for Health announced that community care has failed, many would say that it had never been tried. There is a chance now to turn the concept into reality.

Social work is the profession which looks at the individual in their family and social environment and tries to marshal the resources in those communities to meet the needs of the individual.
mental health services manager, county social services department.

Social work is about people and the identification of the areas which impact on their ability to lead an ordinary life despite their illness.
social worker in mental health services.

Cash versus kind

The legislation and policy guidance around direct payments – Community Care (Direct Payments) Act 1996 – is the latest version of this theme, with its aim to empower those who need services to decide and purchase for their specific requirements.

Information on welfare rights is one of the main issues on which service users' value social work assistance (see Macdonald and Sheldon, 1997).

Liberty versus safety

The philosophical basis of English jurisprudence places a very high emphasis on the liberty of the individual citizen. Philosophical writing such as those of Locke work on liberty, were however, counterbalanced by Hobbes, who argued for a ceding of some freedom of the individual into the power of the state in order to secure their individual and collective safety.

Mental Health is an area where the dichotomy between liberty and safety is most keenly felt. Again, Jones's work is particularly helpful here in demonstrating how political campaigns, notably by the Earl of Shaftesbury in the 19th century, cause célèbres, literature, philosophical thought and financial considerations shape law and practice not in a straight line but rather a series of overlapping circles!

The pendulum is still swinging, with the concerns over the diagnosis of dangerous people with severe personality disorders influencing, some would say over-influencing, the work towards the framing of a replacement of the 1983 Mental Health Act (see Stanley and Manthorpe, 2001, and the Sainsbury Centre for Mental Health, Executive Briefing No. 14, March 2001).

Defining community

Lastly in this section, it is vital that we are very careful in our definitions of 'Community'. Words and concepts tend to have a time-limited and limiting lifespan. A word is used, and indeed often overused, because it has a positive 'feel' to it, and promoted because it can be spoken of almost as a 'good' in itself. Because of lack of definition, and over-utilisation, the word

Figure 3: An historical path – local authority responsibilities.

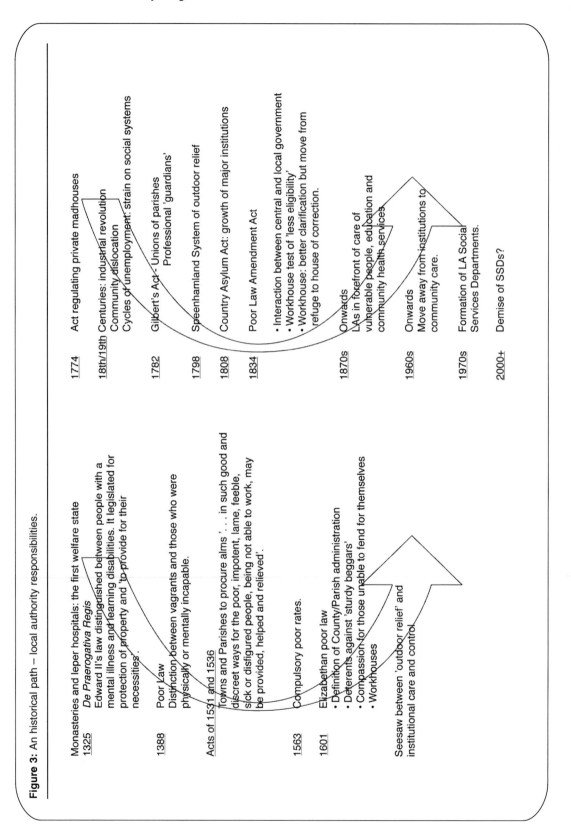

Monasteries and leper hospitals: the first welfare state
1325   *De Praerogativa Regis*
        Edward II's law distinguished between people with a
        mental illness and learning disabilities. It legislated for
        protection of property and 'to provide for their
        necessities'.

1388   Poor Law
        Distinction between vagrants and those who were
        physically or mentally incapable.

Acts of 1531 and 1536
        Towns and Parishes to procure alms ' . . . in such good and
        discreet ways for the poor, impotent, lame, feeble,
        sick or disfigured people, being not able to work, may
        be provided, helped and relieved'.

1563   Compulsory poor rates.

1601   Elizabethan poor law
        • Definition of County/Parish administration
        • Deterrents against 'sturdy beggars'
        • Compassion for those unable to fend for themselves
        • Workhouses

Seesaw between 'outdoor relief' and
institutional care and control

1774   Act regulating private madhouses

18th/19th Centuries: industrial revolution
        Community dislocation
        Cycles of unemployment: strain on social systems

1782   Gilbert's Act - Unions of parishes
                            Professional 'guardians'

1798   Speenhamland System of outdoor relief

1808   Country Asylum Act: growth of major institutions

1834   Poor Law Amendment Act

        • Interaction between central and local government
        • Workhouse test of "less eligibility'
        • Workhouse: better clarification but move from
          refuge to house of correction.

1870s   Onwards
        LAs in forefront of care of
        vulnerable people, education and
        community health services

1960s   Onwards
        Move away from institutions to
        community care.

1970s   Formation of LA Social
        Services Departments.

2000+   Demise of SSDs?

then falls into desuetude or disgrace. Community, especially in the phrase 'Care in the Community' has attracted this special status, and then the resulting opprobrium.

This has most unfortunate consequences because community and its companion words: common (as in the common good), communion, communication, commonwealth etc., have a strong provenance in English language and practical philosophy, and we don't actually have anything better to denote what we mean by groups of people bound together by some form of common interest (see below).

With the growth of communitarian ideas, and a belief that in aspects of education, crime and disorder and the care of vulnerable people, positive communities play a vital part in balancing the interests of individuals, groups and the state at large.

In Peter Bates and David Morris's ground-breaking publication, *Working for Inclusion* (Bates and Morris, 2002), Alyson McCollam and Julia White give the following definitions of community:

- Communities based on geographical areas or neighbourhoods where people live.
- Communities which centre on shared interest or identity (ethnicity, sexuality, faith etc.).
- Areas of shared experiences and feelings leading to 'a sense of community', in addition to the social networks and patterns of behaviour that sustain them.
- Fellowship of interests e.g. those of intellect, philosophy, faith or profession, which reach across geographical boundaries.

Issues that remain are:

- Communities that are created for administrative convenience may receive very little ownership from the citizens they exist to serve. Examples of this would be some of the local authority areas such as Cleveland and Avon, set up in the 1970s and since dismantled under the last round of local government reorganisation. Primary care groups in county areas, which served groups of people around district council boundaries, have since been absorbed into primary care trusts, serving much larger areas, akin to the old district health authority areas, and may now have more clout but less ownership.
- Choice versus ascribed belonging: people may decide to be part of a community. McCollam and White point out that people with mental

health needs are increasingly regarded as part of the wider disability movement but may not perceive themselves as such.
- *Being* in a community versus *being active* in a community: people who live in an area do not necessarily wish to become active. On the other hand, someone who joins a local pressure group, political party etc., may do so in order to campaign on a specific issue or issues.

Events in Northern Ireland, especially those recent happenings in West Belfast around access to schools, and the riots in Oldham and Bradford should caution us as to any romanticised notion of community. Communities can be mutually antagonistic towards each other and can also be closed as well as open and inclusive. 'A distinguishing feature may be the extent to which communities can combine a capacity to maintain internal cohesion with a capacity to be outward looking and sustain links that can reach outside' (McCollam and White, in Bates, 2002).

It is also worth defining the two major uses of 'community' in recent Social and Health Care policy:

- **Community Care** – means planning and providing the services and support which people who are affected by challenges of ageing, mental health needs, learning disability or physical/sensory disability need to be able to live as independently as possible in their own homes, or in 'homely' settings in the community, through the operation of the *National Health Service and Community Care Act 1990* (implemented 1ST April 1993).
- **Care in the community** – the movement of vulnerable adults from long-stay institutions to services – or an absence of services – in community settings. This policy commenced with legislation such as the *1959 Mental Health Act* and the new direction on care given by the Ministry of Health in 1961/62.

I started the chapter with the famous quotation from Margaret Thatcher. In the autumn of 2002, the Conservative Party rode back from this proposition and declared that there is indeed an entity called 'society'.

Images of deviance and difference; policy and legislation; models of care; community relationships, don't take place in a vacuum. Individual health and well-being takes place within a wider context in which we are all a

part. As Plato pointed out, at a time when
human kind was attempting to define civil and
civilised life, there is an inner principle, a goal of
social and individual life working itself out in
society.

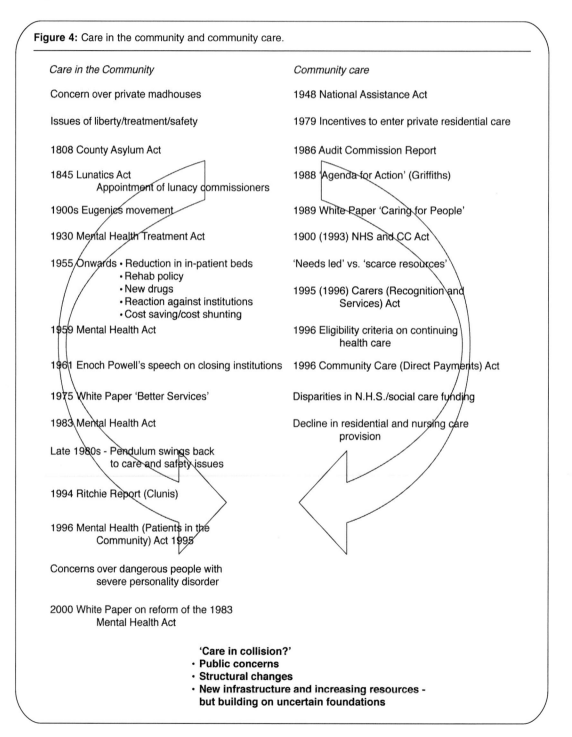

Figure 4: Care in the community and community care.

Care in the Community	Community care
Concern over private madhouses	1948 National Assistance Act
Issues of liberty/treatment/safety	1979 Incentives to enter private residential care
1808 County Asylum Act	1986 Audit Commission Report
1845 Lunatics Act Appointment of lunacy commissioners	1988 'Agenda for Action' (Griffiths)
1900s Eugenics movement	1989 White Paper 'Caring for People'
1930 Mental Health Treatment Act	1900 (1993) NHS and CC Act
1955 Onwards • Reduction in in-patient beds • Rehab policy • New drugs • Reaction against institutions • Cost saving/cost shunting	'Needs led' vs. 'scarce resources'
1959 Mental Health Act	1995 (1996) Carers (Recognition and Services) Act
1961 Enoch Powell's speech on closing institutions	1996 Eligibility criteria on continuing health care
1975 White Paper 'Better Services'	1996 Community Care (Direct Payments) Act
1983 Mental Health Act	Disparities in N.H.S./social care funding
Late 1980s - Pendulum swings back to care and safety issues	Decline in residential and nursing care provision
1994 Ritchie Report (Clunis)	
1996 Mental Health (Patients in the Community) Act 1995	
Concerns over dangerous people with severe personality disorder	
2000 White Paper on reform of the 1983 Mental Health Act	

'Care in collision?'
- **Public concerns**
- **Structural changes**
- **New infrastructure and increasing resources - but building on uncertain foundations**

Chapter 3

Mental Health – At the Heart of Reform

Mental Health – a priority

Drivers for change come from coalitions of implements and power who recognise and express dissatisfaction with the status quo. Concern over the abuses in private 'madhouses' created the impetus to commence the tide of legislation in the 19th century. The failures of the British Army in the Boer War brought about a national debate concerning education, public health, diet and fitness. Pollution and disease spreading to housing areas of all classes in Victorian England led to public health campaigns and the municipalisation of public utilities.

The fact that so many people with mental illness and learning disabilities were removed from their communities (see Jones, 1972; Porter, 2002; Wright and Digby, 1996; Gilbert and Scragg, 1992) meant that services were:

- stigmatised
- separated from community services and networks of all kinds
- poorly resourced
- under-influenced by developments elsewhere

When the institutions were re-labelled as 'hospitals', following the NHS Act of 1946 (implemented 1948), it gave rise to a comforting belief that health care generally and medical care in particular was of a high quality. Anybody having worked in one of the hospitals, however, and all the feedback from community staff regarding the health of patients assessed once they were discharged from a medium or long stay in hospital, tends to show that this was anything but so.

So many of the old institutions have now closed that it is sometimes difficult to convey to new students in medicine, nursing, social work and therapies, the true nature of institutional care. Those who have will immediately recognise the then Minister of Health Enoch Powell's speech in 1961 when he initiated the forthcoming Hospital Plan and the beginning of the closure of the long stay hospitals:

This is a colossal undertaking, not so much in the physical provision which it involves as in the sheer inertia of mind and matter which it requires to be overcome. There they stand, isolated, majestic, imperi-ous, brooded over by the gigantic water tower and chimney combined, rising unmistakable and daunting out of the countryside – the asylums which our forefathers built with such immense solidity. Do not for a moment underestimate their power of resistance to our assault.

quoted in Jones, 1972: p321–2.

As Powell so powerfully puts it, it is cultural rather than physical change which is so hard both to initiate and to sustain.

Mental health is now one of the Government's three stated priorities for the NHS, along with cancer and heart disease. This new focus on mental health is in part due to a realisation that, in an age where the economic strength of the workforce lies in the creativity and intelligence of each individual (see Goleman,1996; Scott, 2001) sound mental health and rapid recovery from mental distress is in the nation's interest. It is the same scale of realisation and political imperative as that over physical health during the Boer War when the effect of poor physical capacity on the Army and industrial production became evident.

Reasons to be cheerful:

- Mental health is now one of the Government's three main health priorities.
- There is a National Director for Mental Health with a Head of Mental Health Services at the Department of Health.
- There is recognition that while specific attention has to be given to those with severe and enduring mental illness, a 'whole systems' approach is required to radically improve the health of the nation.
- The first National Service Framework for a major service in the UK was for mental health.
- A major development of the policy infrastructure and work, which links policy and practice, such as the Care Programme Approach (CPA).
- A greater involvement of a wide range of service users in a way that challenges policy and service delivery at a national, regional and local level. The introduction of NSF 'Framework Champions'. This is allied to legislation such as around direct payments, designed to empower individuals in creating their own service around their specific needs.

- A greater involvement of carers; an approach accelerated following the implementation of the Carers' (Recognition and Services) Act of 1995. While it is recognised that the needs and desires of users may be distinct from their carers, there is great benefit in looking at where the needs are congruent and where they are divergent and being explicit at both an individual and a policy level. Local authorities and their productive links with voluntary and charitable organisations may reasonably be said to have led on this ahead of the NHS.
- Considerable attention given to workforce issues, through the work of the Workforce Action Team, and the benefits of this now beginning to be seen.
- The creation of the National Institute for Mental Health in England (NIMHE, which connects research, good practice and development within a 'Whole Systems' approach.
- The strength of the independent policy centres within the United Kingdom and their ability to appropriately both stand together with and stand to one side of statutory bodies.
- A framework which connects and involves users, carers, practitioners, managers and policy makers at national, regional and local levels through Local Implementation Teams (LITs) Framework Champions, development centres (national and local) etc.
- The building of positive relationships with voluntary, not for profit and private organisations.
- Major investment in mental health services over the next three years, with growth in early intervention, primary care, assertive outreach, support to carers, work in prisons and training.
- Work to reform the 1983 Mental Health Act, and other legislation around human rights, recognition of and support for carers, direct payments etc.
- An underpinning set of values and a recognition of the needs of special attention to race, gender, culture and faith, sexual orientation etc.

Department of Health, 2001.

Reasons to be cautious:

- There is a huge structural change going on in the NHS with 'Shifting the Balance of Power' moving the locus of commissioning to primary care trusts, and seeing the creation of four health and social care regions and strategic health authorities.

- The creation of large mental health trusts and the transfer of general community staff to PCTs may increase the focus on mental health but could lead to their isolation from mainstream influences within the NHS and local authorities.
- The creation of care trusts and the general tendency to transfer local authority functions to the NHS could see a marginalisation of public health expertise and perspective, and a loss of the connectedness with the social inclusion, regeneration, education and citizenship agendas.
- *There seems to be little understanding that the social situation of a person has so much impact on their mental health. There is no point in giving someone medication if they live in condemned accommodation with no heat or water. Medical input is actually a very small part of the overall treatment plan of the client presenting with mental health problems* (social worker in a community team).
- Fears over the 'democratic deficit' and a de-coupling from the democratic process.
- The movement of social work and social care staff to mental health trusts may encourage a re-emergence of a 'medical model' of care and neglect of the social elements which make up the predominant proportion of the concerns of those who use the service (see Chapter 4 below).
- Values, knowledge and skills may become submerged.
- *In an increasingly medical model of community care, it is essential that social workers remain able to provide person-centred and social explanations for a range of behaviours which may otherwise become diagnostic categories* (social worker in a mental health setting).
- The laudable approach to frameworks in education, health and social services has sometimes seen an oppressive increase in bureaucratic procedures and paperwork, resulting in a major loss in direct contact with users and carers.
- The revised guidance of the CPA in 1999 recognises this. It brought in two levels of complexity (standard and enhanced) and required an amalgamation with social services care management procedures.
- *We have to fill in the multi-disciplinary forms which are long but useful for users and ourselves in care planning, but then we have to duplicate it all on the SSD forms!* (social worker in a CMHT, 1996).

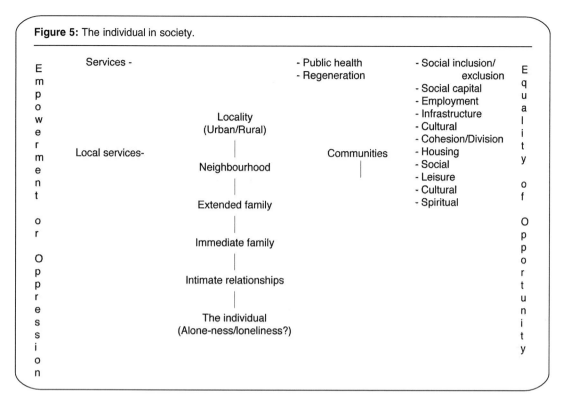

Figure 5: The individual in society.

The developing policy agenda

In line with sound management thinking, the Department of Health has set in place a policy and practice framework through:

- White Paper, *Modernising Mental Health Services* (1998).
- *The National Service Framework for Mental Health* (September 1999).
- The mental health chapter in the *National Health Service Plan*.
- *The Mental Health Policy Implementation Guidance* (2000-ongoing).
- *The Journey to Recovery* (November 2001).
- *Making it Happen: A Guide to Delivering Mental Health Promotion* (May 2001).

The Implementation guide has specific sections on:

- crisis resolution
- assertive outreach
- early intervention
- primary care
- health promotion
- tailoring service to local needs
- achieving and securing progress

Further policies are being developed on:

- women and mental health
- mental health and people from black and ethnic minorities (for spring 2003)

Mental health within a wider context

If we accept that individuals live and work within a variety of relationships, networks and environments, then we must increasingly orientate ourselves towards a holistic and 'whole systems' approach.

As Peter Bates puts it in his introduction to the SCMH pack on social inclusion:

> *The more work we gathered together the more it became clear that social inclusion was not merely an attractive goal for mental health services – it was imperative.*
>
> SCMH, 2002: p3. (my emphasis)

Mental health services, because of the individualised, medical approach enshrined in the UK since the mid/late 19th century, still tend to concentrate on individual pathology. But the individual originates from some form of family or substitute family context; may well live with a partner; as part of an extended family; and be or have dependents.

Assessment, treatment, care, support and rehabilitation has to take place within a context of neighbourhoods, groups and communities, and the policies of public health, regeneration, political priorities (both national and local) will have a major impact on the meaning individuals have in their lives, and the environment in which they try and function.

The revised CPA Guidance makes it clear that:

Evidence and experiences demonstrated the benefits of well co-ordinated care to those with Mental Health problems. Mental health service users, particularly those with the most complex and enduring needs, can require help with other aspects of their lives, e.g. housing, finance, employment, education and physical health needs. Mental illness places demands on services that no one discipline or agency can meet alone.

p2.

Stanley and Manthorpe, in their review of the major mental health enquiries, comment both that, in the case of Stephen Laudat 'Mainstream agencies often fail to accept the contribution that can be made by families and communities.' (Stanley and Manthorpe, 2001: p89).

And again:

The enquiry team examining the care of Anthony Smith identified the failure of the team to address his problems of unemployment and housing which were likely to contribute to a relapse . . . the focus was on treating the illness rather than the patient in the round.

quoted in Stanley and Manthorpe, 2001: p92.

Social work is about people and identification of the areas which impact on their ability to lead an ordinary life despite their illness.

social worker.

It was with increasing recognition that social and environmental aspects of mental health were increasingly important, and a growing concern that the medical model might be inappropriately reasserted, that led to the formation of the Social Perspectives Network in the autumn of 2001. Work within the network redefined the social model in mental health and set out the following characteristics of it as follows:

- It is based on an understanding of complexity of human health and well-being.
- It emphasises the interaction of social factors with those of biology and microbiology in construction of health and disease.
- It addresses the inner and outer worlds of individuals, groups and communities.
- It embraces the experiences and supports the social networks of people who are vulnerable and frail.

- It understands and works collaboratively within the institutions of civil society to promote the interests of individuals and communities and can also critique and challenge where these are detrimental to those interests.
- It emphasises shared knowledge and shared territory with a range of disciplines and with service users and the general public.
- It emphasises empowerment and capacity building at individual and community level and therefore tolerates and celebrates difference.
- It places equal value on the expertise of service users, carers and the general public but will challenge attitudes and practices that are oppressive, judgemental and destructive.
- It operationalises a critical understanding of the nature of power and hierarchy in the creation of health inequalities and social inclusion.
- It is committed to the development of theory and practice and the critical evaluation of process and outcome.

Duggan with Foster and Cooper, 2002.

The ancient code of Hamurabi (1728–1686 BC) stated that you cannot separate the illness from the patient. Some centuries on, it is clear that one cannot separate the illness from the individual, the family, the community or the health of the nation.

Changing structures

'Form follows function' is a useful dictum, and yet there sometimes appears to be an obsession with structural change as the way of resolving a range of challenges. In fact, of course, there is usually an excellent rationale for any reconfiguration of organisational structures. In the NHS for example:

- Area Health Authorities – with their coterminosity with county councils made a great deal of sense in the 1970s.
- District Health Authorities – created 'to bring the NHS closer to the people'.
- The purchaser/provider split (as opposed to the purchaser/provider *separation* in local authorities) – 'to bring the discipline of the market into the NHS'. Except, it became in most cases 'playing shops' with an increase in paper exchange resulting in little discernible change in behaviours.

- Primary care groups – set up to involve GPs – benefit from the experience of fundholding and total purchasing projects, and create synergies with district councils and their environmental health responsibilities.
- Primary care trusts – to form larger commissioning bodies with a primary care focus, but with a possibility of losing the local responsiveness created by PCGs.
- Care trusts to bring the NHS and social care together and tear down 'the Berlin wall' between these two major agencies. The model is based on that which is said to work well in Northern Ireland, except that a closer examination shows an all too familiar pattern in the Province of domination by acute hospitals and neglect of some vital social care perspectives (see Campbell and McLaughlin, 2000).

All these models have a great deal of merit in themselves. But there is an insistent restlessness which leads to headlines such as: 'April again?: Time for another reorganisation'. (*Health Service Journal*, 4th April 2002) and the impression of a search for a structural nirvana.

Reorganisations in terms of structural change and/or mergers in public or private organisations tend to:

'Suck up a lot of management time, and that's not just manager managers but clinical managers as well', Matt Tee, Communications Director, Commission for Health Improvement (CHI) (quoted in *Health Service Journal*, 14th February 2002).

Encourage people to look inwards rather than outwards.

There is a heightened risk that the eye gets taken off the ball of service delivery
> Tim Matthews, former Chief Executive of St Thomas's Hospital, who steered through its merger with Guys Hospital in 1993 (quoted in *HSJ*, 14th February 2002).

In fact, there is no structural 'Emerald City'. In the end, like Dorothy, we have to stop relying on the Wizards of Oz, or Whitehall, and work more co-operatively together on a common agenda, forged through discussion and co-operation. Ultimately, it is *people* who drive positive change, not structures.

Social work values are directly at odds with the organisation that I am soon going to have to be employed by.
> social worker contemplating working within a combined health and social care trust.

You have to keep re-asserting the local authority agenda.
> member of a community mental health team for older people, quoted in SSI/Audit Commission, Dec. 2001.

In this diagram the source of power and decision-making 'A', makes rulings and sends out instructions. Limited discussion and modification is made by senior managers at 'B', but real power remains with the central caucus. Middle managers at 'C' have no real power to influence events and are the rotating arm of the module or the chain attached to the hammer, and can therefore only try and keep in touch with both staff and higher management. Staff at 'D' are subject to the full velocity of change with all the sense of potential helplessness and disillusion which that implies.

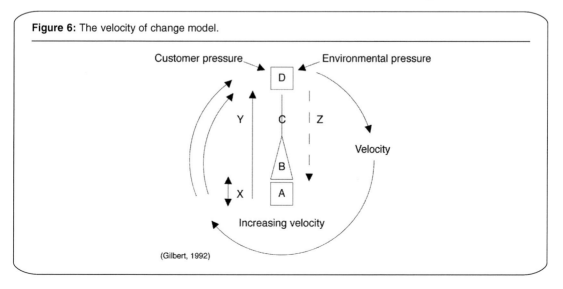

Figure 6: The velocity of change model.

(Gilbert, 1992)

The real interchange of ideas only takes place at 'X' with the directive proceeding along line 'Y'. Disinformation, and environmental and customer pressures has a modifying effect at the customer interface 'D', and this is fed back slowly along line 'Z'. The time-lag and the power energy at the centre means that 'A' is already generating new ideas that have to be passed down the line and implemented before the first batch have been properly bedded down. The middle management process tends to get stretched and collapsed like a piece of elastic and often loses its coherence and creativity.

Mental health services are moving towards various forms of integration. When in 1996 Somerset Health Authority and County Councils reviewed their mental health services, the experiences of users led them to set up a Joint Commissioning Board and combined service provision (see Gulliver, Peck and Towell, June 2000, August 2000, February 2001). Chris Davies, Director of Social Services for Somerset, has remarked that he attracted some criticism from fellow social services directors at the time for 'handing services from the local authority to the NHS'. But Davies felt strongly that with mental health services being only about eight per cent of the social services budget, the social care perspective, broader local authority agenda and public health issues were better championed by an integrated approach rather than continued separation, even though the provision of service in effect went into a health agency. It was perhaps helpful that the first chief executive of the Somerset Partnership Trust was someone with a social work training and background.

Since the mid-1990s, arrangements like Somerset have become increasingly more common through the flexibilities under Section 31 of the 1999 Health Act, and on the 1st April 2002, three care trusts, focusing on users with mental health needs, were launched in Manchester, Bradford and Camden and Islington.

In the eastern region, a working group has looked specifically at 'adding value to mental health partnership organisations through the successful integration of social care', (Modernisation Taskforce Report, 27th February 2002). The partnership members have recognised that 'service users and carers value services that are influenced significantly by the 'social model of disability/disadvantage', comparing such services very favourably against any experiences that they consider to be over-influenced by a traditional 'medical model''. Progressive medical practitioners recognise this and thus it is vital to understand and benefit from:

- Understanding the NHS inheritance. The NHS's familiarity with internal integration issues both organisationally and clinically.
- The importance of social perspectives especially within the wider agenda of community capacity building, employment, housing and social groups.

The working group have identified a number of specific valued elements the Social Care tradition brings to Mental Health.

'It is noticeable', says the document, 'that many of these characteristics seem essential to achieving National Service Framework standards'.

Table 1: Distinctive strength of the mental health social care tradition.

- Specialist social work responsibilities since 1959 and accumulated experience.
- Needs-led assessment and care management since 1993, and their contribution to the holistic implementation of the care programme approach.
- An emphasis on the preferences and choices of individual service users and carers (sometimes summarised as 'the social work approach'). The most recent example is facilitating this through 'direct payments'.
- Specific developments in recognition and support for carers – including the separate assessment of carers' needs.
- Support for advocacy services.
- Initiatives in involving service users and carers (or their representatives) in consultation and service planning.
- Service developments in social care support for people with mental health problems.
- Strong associations with the 'social model' of disability/disadvantage and the overall social inclusion agenda.
- Positive record on anti-discriminatory services and promoting the needs of ethnic minority communities and disabled people etc.
- Part of the wider council tradition of community development.
- Good links with employment, leisure and – especially – housing services through being part of local authorities.
- A strong tradition of staff supervision and training.

The series of evaluation articles on the Somerset experience, which have run in *Managing Community Care* (see Gulliver, Peck and Towell, op cit) show that, despite clear leadership from the top, structural integration and the concomitant development of inter-professional co-operation to produce better outcomes for service users and carers requires considerable ongoing application. While the most consistent aspiration voiced by senior managers and local politicians for the formation of the combined trust, was the creation of a 'seamless service' supported by 'shared culture', the staff surveys picked up some lack of certainties around organisational identity and strategic direction; some uncertainty around professional roles and personal skills; and increased pressures. On the positive side, there appeared to be greater cohesion amongst the staff group; increased clarity about the teams' task; a greater appreciation of each other's professional roles and being involved in joint assessments; and an appreciation of the greater variety of work.

Within this mixed picture, with progress clearly being made, the authors make the point that:

'Co-location and revised management arrangements may not in themselves be sufficient to develop 'shared culture' and enhance 'shared working', and that the trust may have to adopt some further strategies for change'. (Gulliver et al., 2001.)

Change is a long-term process. Changing the structures is relatively easy; changing the culture takes time and attention. John P. Kotter, in his incisive article on why efforts to transform organisations can so easily fail, suggests that 'declaring victory too soon' and not 'anchoring changes in the organisation's culture', are two major reasons for failure. (Kotter, 1995.) I have recently produced a ten-point change process, adapted from Kotter's eight-point scale, and others, including Proehl's consideration of public sector organisations, and this has the following stages:

1. Determining the need for change.
2. Establishing a sense of urgency.
3. Creating the guiding coalition.
4. Developing a vision and strategy.
5. Communicating the change vision.
6. Working with the human factors.
7. Empowering broad-based action.
8. Generating short-term wins.
9. Consolidating gains and producing more change.
10. Anchoring new approaches in the culture.
    Gilbert, 2003/4, forthcoming, adapted from Kotter, 1995, and Proehl, 2001.

'On an encouraging note, the Manchester Care Trust, with its history of partnership previous to April 2002, has seen a reduction in emergency hospital admissions over a three-month period, down from 16 per cent to eight per cent, a 22 to thirty per cent increase in the number of clients with intensive care needs supported in the community rather than in residential placements, and a halving in waiting times to see a consultant'. (George, April 2002.) Increased involvement of service users and carers in the planning and delivery of services is also quoted as an advantage in the Manchester Model as is their participation in training programmes, including those for psychiatrists. In the inner city of Camden and Islington 'the main advantage is seen as the care trust's ability to make social inclusion its 'core business'', (George, April 2002).

The study by Macdonald and Sheldon in Westminster in the late 1990s reinforced the need for a social perspective:

Of the 92 clients interviewed, 85% survived on income support. A further seven (8%) received invalidity benefit . . . Most (71%) lived in rented accommodation; with a further 21% in hostel accommodation. 87% were unemployed. Socio-economic factors are known to play a significant part in the ability of clients to cope with mental illness and the pressures which they signify are good predictors of the need for services and their influence on relapse rates.
                    Macdonald and Sheldon, 1997.

At the end of the day, the acid test for structural change has to be improved outcomes for service users and carers.

For the last three years she has been there whether it is for practical issues, medical issues, or just a shoulder to cry on. I feel there have been times when, without the support and understanding of the social worker, I would not have coped. It has been a lifeline to me and has helped me make progress through some very difficult experiences.
                    Leeds Consumer Survey, January, 1997.

There is a great deal to be encouraged about in mental health services today, but it is also too easy for managers, practitioners, those involved in governance and services as a whole to become side-tracked or pre-occupied by factors which are not the core issues for the service: e.g. structures, targets which are not well focused, inter-disciplinary rivalries etc. The leadership role for practitioners and managers is to keep their sights set firmly on core values and core goals.

Chapter 4

Society is Us! – The Service User's View

*When I think what he said on Tuesday – 'leave the medication to me. I'll make the decisions on that. That's why you chose me as your psychiatrist'. ---- off, Graham, it should be a partnership. We have to arrive at decisions with negotiation. **He** doesn't have to take the drugs. If I'm not in agreement, when this section is lifted, I won't co-operate. This all sounds very childish. Perhaps it's just Graham's attitude which makes me cross but then he puts me in a powerless position. I hate all psychiatrists, all registrars, all nurses, cleaners, cooks, managers, community psychiatric nurses and Virginia Bottomley.*

> Linda Hart, *Phone at Nine Just to Say You're Alive*, 1997.

The system hasn't ever been designed around the patient, whereas almost every business these days is having to design itself around whatever you call them – customers or clients or whatever.

> Derek Wanless, author of The Wanless Report on the NHS (*HSJ*, 25.4.2002).

The one thing that would have made a difference, I think, would have been someone to talk to (on admission to psychiatric hospital). That was what I was always wondering, when I went into hospital: would there be someone to talk to? But I used to shut myself off. Maybe if depression had been explained to me earlier . . .

Annemarie Randall, *The Observer*, 7th April 2002.

In the debate about different models of care:

> *. . . let us be proactive and not reactive. Let's reclaim the evidence with and for the service users. It all comes from service users anyway in the first place. Let's find out what service users say or have already said about what works and is helpful and let's spread this evidence throughout the land.*

> Thurstine Bassett, independent consultant and trainer, personal communication, May, 2002.

Without medication, we would both put our heads in the gas oven. We couldn't cope at all without social workers with all the stress and problems in our lives.

> service user quoted in Macdonald and Sheldon, 1997.

It is difficult for front line staff to walk around with a lot of performance indicators in their heads. In inducting new staff when I was chief executive of a trust, I would simply ask them to have in their heads the constant question: 'would this service be good enough for me or my family?'

> Christina Pond, NHS Leadership Centre (conversation with author).

One of the worst days of my life, but I have been loved by Margaret and Basil, Gordon, Sheila, Annie, Rita, Joy, Kate and Jane, Jack and William . . .

> Linda Hart, op cit.

Surely it would be good to have a cup of tea and a welcome into a frightening environment.

> service user quoted in NHS Modernisation Agency, *Mental Health Pilot: Improvement Case Studies*, DoH, 2002.

I don't remember his name or have ever seen him since the thirty minutes he spent with me fifteen years ago but his message of hope he gave me has never left.

> service user, quoted in *Developing a Recovery Platform for Mental Health Service Delivery for People with Mental Illness/Distress in England*, 2002.

Only connect

Having worked in both learning disability and mental health services, I find it fascinating that issues of citizenship and empowerment appear to be much more firmly embedded in the culture of the former than in the latter, and in many ways there appears to be a greater belief in the developmental progress that people with learning disabilities can make than in the field of mental health where the Recovery movement is having to combat considerable prejudice, both latent and overt.

Both the Mental Health White Paper and policy documents, and the White Paper on Learning Disabilities (NIMHE Consultation Document, June 2001, *The Journey to Recovery*, November, 2001, *Valuing People*, March 2001, Mental Health White Paper, *Modernising Mental Health Services*, 1998), emphasise that services must be built on:

- The legal and civil rights of service users and carers.
- The innate dignity of each individual.
- Respect for cultural and ethnic diversity.
- The centrality of user involvement in the care planning and delivery process.
- Accessibility of services and choice.
- Working in partnership to produce the right outcomes for people, based on their existing support networks – both personal and community.

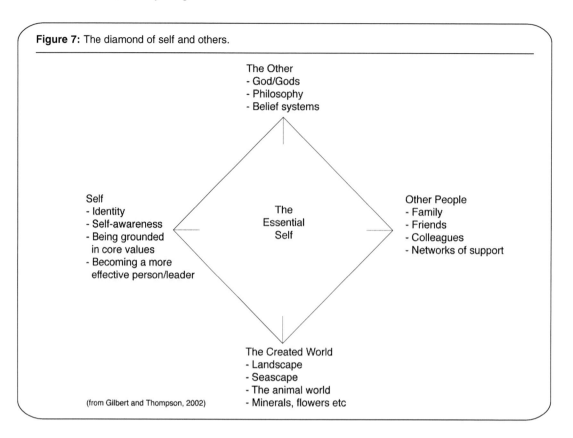

Figure 7: The diamond of self and others.

The Other
- God/Gods
- Philosophy
- Belief systems

Self
- Identity
- Self-awareness
- Being grounded
  in core values
- Becoming a more
  effective person/leader

The
Essential
Self

Other People
- Family
- Friends
- Colleagues
- Networks of support

The Created World
- Landscape
- Seascape
- The animal world
- Minerals, flowers etc

(from Gilbert and Thompson, 2002)

• Respect for staff and their needs as the service can only fundamentally exist in relationships between people.

*Feedback must not only be a task but a **value** held through all stages of service provision. Feedback must be mutual, not excluding service users, individual service provision, general comments about services that promote constructive comments and complements. An environment must cultivate feedback as integral to developing responsive service delivery.*
    document on recovery, (draft, 6th March 2002).

The longer I live the more I believe that real life is about our connectedness with other people, with 'the other' (whatever that is, and it means many different things to different people) and other aspects of life.

Mental distress and mental illness is so often about a disconnection, false connections or an over-concentration on one aspect of our lives. As a runner, for example, I know that dedicating a certain amount of time to the sport helps my general fitness and alertness; gives me a 'high' through the release of endorphins; connects me to the landscapes and seascapes

I'm running through; and provides a bond with other runners. I am also aware that it can become an obsession; the need for 'a fix', the minutiae of race times, over-competitiveness etc.

The actress Nicola Pagett in her moving description of a manic depressive illness writes that:

Everything was unbearably, unutterably beautiful. I didn't need my husband any more. There were the cameras to talk to and the radio people to take care of me . . . I've always known what love is ever since I was small. I've always known it was for better or worse but I forgot. I pushed them away, those who love me, my husband and my daughter. I hardly spoke to them and when I did, it was brusque, clipped. They weren't real, I couldn't see them, there was something in the way and they wouldn't let me listen to my music. It didn't seem loud to me.
    Nicola Pagett, *Diamonds Behind my Eyes*, 1998.

To really engage with service users, and their carers and supporters, we need to be mindful of the 'whole person' within a context of family, neighbourhood and community; their history, hopes, fears and aspirations; and the strengths and needs they bring to the table.

Figure 8: Starting from the user's perspective.

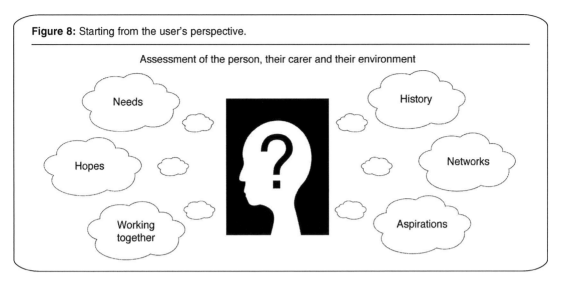

Assessment of the person, their carer and their environment

Needs

History

Hopes

Networks

Working together

Aspirations

Quite simply, social workers have the wider view, which is particularly important for those having difficulty in engaging with services and society.
consultant psychiatrist with special expertise in working with people with personality disorders.

The value of social work in the provision of modern mental health services must be a particular understanding of people in the context of their lives and communities.
Director of Social Care in a mental health NHS trust (from a nursing and health policy background).

The word 'assessment' comes from the Latin, 'assidere' – 'to sit beside' someone, and it is only by getting alongside of the person we are trying to serve that we can release their own innate capacity to find themselves, regain control over their lives and move forward on their previous road or in exploring fresh avenues.

There may be a tendency to think that empowerment is all about middle class aspirants who have suffered some temporary disruption in their lives, but participation and self-fulfilment are crucial aspects wherever we start the journey, whatever path we are on and wherever we are going to.

Case Example 2

'Arnold' had a diagnosis of severe and enduring mental illness. He had become very socially isolated, with a history of non-compliance with social and medical intervention, and many previous admissions to hospital.

In looking at the whole picture of Arnold's life: his style of life in an isolated rural community, with little formal education and no friends, meant that he lacked confidence and self-esteem.

Following discussion with Arnold, and in liaison with his carer, and colleagues within the multi-disciplinary team, the social worker involved a community support worker who began weekly visits to support Arnold in his daily living skills and also worked with him in attending a social drop-in centre.

As Arnold's confidence built up, shopping trips were added and other social activities. A separate assessment of the needs of Arnold's carer was completed under the Carer's (Recognition and Services) Act 1995 and support was established with the local carer support service.

The close and regular input from the community support worker has enabled Arnold to engage with services more positively, increase social contacts, develop self-confidence and new skills, so that he can continue to live in the community without further hospital admissions to date; and it is has also ensured support for the carer so as to prevent a breakdown of that vital relationship.

Case Example 3

For many years it was considered the day hospital was vital to me staying alive. Having constant observation was a comfort to those that supported me. I learned very quickly that I was someone that people had little hope that I could self-direct and participate in a life outside a 'treatment facility'. This very quickly became entrenched as part of my identity, which helped only to contribute to what I understand they call 'revolving door syndrome'.

As coincidence helps change direction, I have been prescribed exercise after a serious operation. I enjoyed exercising and for the first time in a long while I didn't have to identify myself as a mentally ill person. I contacted a trainer to help me when I had trouble motivating myself. I soon found that it was more effective for my mental well-being to replace day hospital with gym sessions. At the gym, I could divert my internal attention to external drive and goals. I reconnected with my ability to achieve at what I put my mind to. I found I could manage many distressing symptoms this way.

Besides my trainer becoming one of my closest friends, she is the person who supports me but does not allow excuses for my illness. **This has been so liberating**.

taken from *Developing a Recovery Platform* (draft) 6th March 2002.

Another myth is that of the inevitable separation of users and staff, as though the former are in the swamp and the latter are far removed on well-intended hillside parkland. On the contrary, many members of staff have experienced a form of mental illness and, of course, most will have experienced a period or periods of mental distress. The trouble is that often service environments do not welcome this kind of sharing. Recently, however, Dr Mike Shooter the incoming (June, 2002) President of the Royal College of Psychiatrists, has spoken movingly on the radio of his depression while in his final year as a medical student, and how vital it was that significant people in his life gave him hope and encouragement. Crucially, his medical supervisor believed that this episode would strengthen his ability to be an effective doctor rather than hinder it.

Whether we have suffered from a mental illness or not, we are all likely to have experienced episodes of mental distress through trauma or life crises. We need to get and keep in touch with what is vulnerable in ourselves – and not be frightened of it – so as to be able to work alongside others in distress.

To see ourselves and other people in a holistic way, it is helpful to view the various facets of our humanity:

- Social/emotional needs:
  - relationships; loving and being loved
  - security
  - acknowledgement and expression of feelings
  - kinship
  - friendships
  - community involvement
  - empathy
  - appreciation of creation
- Mental or cognitive needs:
  - opportunities for fresh thinking
  - reading, and reflection on the texts
  - planning ahead
  - creative writing
  - visualising positive futures
  - professional development
  - films and plays
- Spiritual needs:
  - recommitting to core values
  - gaining a meaning for life
  - exploration of 'being' and 'becoming'
  - meditation and contemplation
- Physical needs:
  - a healthy diet
  - physical fitness
  - a sense of well-being and being better able to cope with the stresses of work
  - gaining a sleep and awake time balance
- Creative needs:
  - using our senses
  - exploring new ways of working/leisure
  - developing creative hobbies
    From Gilbert and Thompson, 2002: p106–7.

Maslow's well known work on 'needs' places these in a hierarchy from the most basic to the most profound.

The basic physical needs are food, water, shelter etc., the components of survival, security and safety needs come into play when our physical needs are satisfied and we seek a protection against danger and deprivation. Once

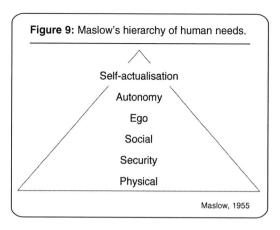

Figure 9: Maslow's hierarchy of human needs.

Self-actualisation

Autonomy

Ego

Social

Security

Physical

Maslow, 1955

we feel secure in ourselves and secure against external threat, we can move into contact with other people in search of friendship, intimacy and a sense of belonging to individuals and groups. Belonging in itself is not usually enough, we are then driven to becoming valued by the people and groups of people we are interacting with in a search for ego strength and esteem. As we become stronger as individuals, we look towards asserting our own individualism and autonomy; and this may well lead on to self-actualisation -a desire to fulfil our potential and talents, even though this sometimes is to the detriment of some of our more basic needs. The recent interest in the explorer Ernest Shackleton in books, films and documentaries is partly a consideration of what drove the Antarctic explorer to place so much at risk to achieve self-actualisation, and his use of the hierarchy of needs in the people he led to attain goals, preserve their safety and keep them together as a team. (See Maslow, 1955, and Cooper and Makin, 1984; for a fascinating insight into Shackleton see Morrell and Capparell, 2001).

Whilst the immediate work with a user may focus on their need to address a place to live, food, treatment and safety; any planning must engage with emotional needs and with aspirations which make life worth living. Mere existence is not enough!

From the identification of need, we move to, as Spicker puts it: 'if people are to make an effective demand for welfare, they have not only to exercise their formal entitlements but also to overcome a series of practical obstacles'.

In all the roles I fulfilled in various social services departments, the desires of users and carers for more and better information was a constant. 'Knowledge is power', as the saying goes, and despite the fact that most statutory

agencies have moved on a long way from the: 'don't let us produce any information otherwise they'll all want some(!)', information is a frequent clarion call. This is particularly true in the case of black and ethnic minorities where the issues are manifestly more complex. One Asian woman caring for her elderly mother with a long history of depressive illness told me that a very well produced leaflet from the London Borough of . . . had come through their front door. It was in the right language but unfortunately the mother could speak the language but not read it, and the daughter could neither speak nor read it fluently. One major element of conscious and unconscious racism in our society is our inability or unwillingness to inform individuals and communities of their rights and their right to services.

Spicker, in his thematic approach to social policy, quotes Kerr in outlining a number of stages that service users have to go through:

- People must feel a need, or at least they must want to have what is being offered.
- They have to find out that the service exists. Even when they have identified their need for something, they may not realise that a service actually exists.
- They have to know that they are likely to receive it. A service which is for 'poor people' is not certain to be taken up by people who do not think of themselves as 'poor'.
- They have to feel that the service/benefit is worth claiming. Sometimes the service is so inflexible that it causes more problems than it solves.
- There are the beliefs and feelings of potential recipients, and as we have seen above, the issue of reciprocity is very important.
- People need to have a sense as to whether the service being offered is likely to help them through a period of time, not just immediately, but that the service may help them over a period of time, or can be adjusted as their needs change. (From Spicker, 1995).

You don't get the information from the staff . . . You either have to rely on other patients to tell you the information, which you might not want to, rely on, or just ignore the whole problem altogether . . . I would have found it much more helpful if someone had actually sat down with me and explained whatever happened to me, how I had got to hospital, what they thought was wrong with me and how they envisage life going for me.
service user quoted in *Mental Health Foundation*, November 1999.

When I was admitted to hospital for a sinus operation, the ward sister sat down with all of us admitted on the same day and explained step by step exactly what was going to happen in terms of care, pre-treatment, the operation and after care. She used simple diagrams and was very happy to field questions. All of us felt much more reassured and in control in an alien environment, and an additional outcome was that we were all very supportive of each other during the whole process.

The Westminster Study

Geraldine Macdonald and Brian Sheldon's 1997 study of people with a mental illness in Westminster and their relationship with their social workers, gives a very clear picture of loss and deprivation in a London borough with high social mobility.

As quoted earlier in this book, 85 per cent of the clients interviewed survived on income support. A further eight per cent received invalidity benefit, and five users reported receiving occasional income from other sources such as training courses. Most (71 per cent) lived in rented accommodation, with a further 21 per cent in hostels. 87 per cent were unemployed, 'socio-economic factors are known to play a significant part in the ability of clients to cope with mental illness and the pressures which they signify are good predictors of the need for services and their influence on relapse rates' (Macdonald and Sheldon, 1997).

Of the kind of problems they experienced, it was the range of interpersonal and social issues which challenge us all, but become especially

Table 2: The incidence of problems cited by respondents.

Problem	N*	%*
Mental state	64	25
Financial difficulties/problems	41	16
Family relationships	25	10
Housing/accommodation	24	9
Social isolation	24	9
Practical problems	22	8
Medical	16	6
Unemployment/boredom	13	5
Living circumstances	11	4
Other	20	8
Total	**260**	**100**

*Respondents often cited more than one problem. Percentages are of the sample interviewed.

hard to overcome when allied with recurrent or chronic illness, and when living in an area where social problems are exacerbated.

The author's remark that '. . . many recurrent problems were social and financial in nature and not *directly* related to the mental condition of the clients'. It is worth noting that while people's mental state was a high preoccupation with the users interviewed, medical issues featured fairly low on the list. It is very evident that the multi-faceted nature of the challenges facing this group and need to broker solutions with a wide range of agencies and community groups were something which played to a specific strength of social work.

Service users were overwhelmingly positive about the work that social workers undertook with them:

* Clients valued the opportunity to discuss and clarify their worries and fears, and examine ways of overcoming them.
* The actual support from a social worker appeared as the most often quoted source of positive services. Next in order of perceived significance were day centres or drop-in facilities, followed by practical help, advocacy and accommodation.
* Most respondents perceived social workers treating them with dignity and respect.
* 60 per cent of those interviewed 'recognised the pivotal role of social workers in providing and co-ordinating services' (Macdonald and Sheldon), though a number felt that their psychiatrist was the central figure.
* Service users appear to feel that the contact they had with social workers was appropriate to their needs.

This kind of feedback is mirrored in the Leeds Survey (Leeds, 1997) where 92 per cent of users who responded identified 'the service of talking, listening, and counselling, as being provided by their social worker'. 75 per cent of respondents considered talking, listening and counselling as being the most beneficial service provided by the social worker.

The next highest figure in this category is advice on benefits. Social workers were seen as dealing with requests adequately (87 per cent); being helpful (96 per cent); and being punctual and reliable (82 per cent).

These services are superb, they help you a lot and without them you'd be sunk.

service user in the Westminster Study.

Figure 10: What service users want.

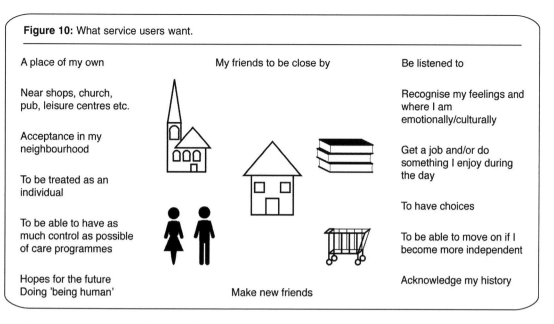

A place of my own	My friends to be close by	Be listened to
Near shops, church, pub, leisure centres etc.		Recognise my feelings and where I am emotionally/culturally
Acceptance in my neighbourhood		Get a job and/or do something I enjoy during the day
To be treated as an individual		To have choices
To be able to have as much control as possible of care programmes		To be able to move on if I become more independent
Hopes for the future Doing 'being human'	Make new friends	Acknowledge my history

I find my social worker excellent, reliable, reassuring, punctual, helpful and genuine.

Always friendly and reliable – always contacts me if unable to see me on the day planned. Good liaison between social worker and doctor.

Living alone, this service is more than important to me having an understanding person to listen to me and give advice in absolute confidence.

service users in the Leeds Survey.

The Westminster Study was not entirely positive, however. Problems identified were:

- Structural gaps between general practitioners and social workers.
- A significant number of service users did not feel that their social workers understood the nature of their problems, or disagreed substantially about their priority. As one service user put it 'He wants to make a life as he sees it. He's not very sympathetic. He speaks in a soft voice to cover up his bad temper and this makes me bad tempered after speaking to him. We are not able to talk'. On the other hand, where differences in perspective were dealt with in a genuine manner, then this was appreciated 'He doesn't always agree about my voices, and says, 'no, it's your sicknesses. I can talk to him about it. I feel quite comfortable discussing differences of opinion with him'.
- There was a lack of choice in the services offered. Almost half felt they had no choice at all *'in the services they use'*.
- One of the most significant findings, and a very disturbing one, was that service users

'were not routinely provided with sufficient opportunities to discuss what was happening to them, nor were they always given information about their legal rights', during compulsory admission to hospital. This will be discussed further in Chapter 6.

Strategies for living

One of the most influential studies in recent times has been the Mental Health Foundation's *Strategies for Living* report of user-led research into people's strategies for living with mental distress and mental illness, published in November 1999.

As the first service user quoted puts it:

We are all primary experts on our own mental health and about what works for us . . . We can and should value the coping strategies we have developed for ourselves . . .

Mental Health Foundation, November 1999.

And the main findings demonstrate:

1. *A demand to be seen as fellow citizens and treated with humanity and dignity.*

Something that is often said by users, carers and frontline staff is 'nobody listens to me!' The concept of citizenship, dating back to the foundations of Western democracy, and in many other non-Euro-centric cultures, is that of the citizen partaking, speaking and being listened to in a public forum. Discussion and debate in the political arena or around the family/community hearth required well-honed listening skills. In modern society, we seem to

Table 3: What was helpful about relationships.

Good relationships gave people:	
Emotional support	*Companionship and friendship*
• acceptance	• shared experiences
• self-acceptance	• shared interests
• understanding	• someone to live for
Meaning	*Practical support*
• sense of belonging	• dealing with professionals
• sense of purpose	• domestic tasks
• someone to live for	• personal care
	• help managing mental health problems
	• financial help

Mental Health Foundation, 1999, p21.

have lost, in many instances, the art of narrative, of telling a story and giving it and the teller space to be valued.

2. *A need to be in as much control as possible of one's diagnosis, treatment and care*.

Linda Hart recalls her psychiatrist changing his mind about her diagnosis 'What peeves me most, is that on the first or second interview I ever had with Graham (the Psychiatrist), I said I was suffering from depression with psychosis and he said, 'no, you're straight down the line, schizophrenic'. Pity these doctors don't listen to their patients' (Hart, 1997, p232).

Of course, being offered a diagnosis and an opportunity to discuss symptoms and causes is usually very helpful 'Yes, it made sense of all the symptoms, but I hadn't thought of it myself . . . It just made sense, not sleeping, waking up early and not being able to get to sleep and not being able to eat, being constantly worried about what was going to happen, that sort of thing'. (A woman on being given a diagnosis of endogenous depression, quoted in Mental Health Foundation, 1999.)

3. *The importance of relationships and informal support*.

Strategies for Living found that about two thirds of their respondents rated the relationships they formed with others as the most important factor in helping them to cope with mental distress.

The study groups the aspects of relationships which people found helpful into four categories (see Table 3):

From my own experience of depression, stemming from work-related stress, I found the following helpful:

• A friend who had been through work-related stress and depression and was able to

empathise with my condition, but also give sound advice from a user perspective on very pertinent matters such as the side effects of anti-depressant medication.

• Friends who were able to give listening time and absorb strong emotions such as anger, pain and anxiety about the future, without feeling overwhelmed.

• People who shared the same spiritual world-view as I did and were able to help me put current events into a wider and deeper perspective.

• A social group who were just generally supportive without needing to have a great deal of understanding about the specific issues.

• People who went through a similar experience of depression who sought my help when I was in recovery – the importance of reciprocity.

• A GP who related to my pain in a very human way and allowed me maximum choice over the timing and type of treatment.

• A friend who recognised the importance of words and wrote me a card describing my qualities as she saw them.

4. *Being able to give as well as to receive*.

Very few of us feel comfortable in a purely receiving mode once we leave childhood. Being a constant recipient feeds into a feeling of powerlessness and losing our rights and responsibilities as citizens.

Some of the most powerful testimonies on this is listening to members of the medical profession who have themselves been recipients of health services.

The following case example demonstrates the upward spiral which can result when people are

Case Example 4

'Julie' was a recently separated mother of four. She suffered with anxiety, clinical depression and a history of self-harm. The two children living at home, both in their mid teens, had been identified as the main carers and involved in all aspects of domestic care. Julie was often incapacitated by her depression and stayed in bed. The community team worked with her to identify a care plan which worked on self-confidence issues, enhancing social opportunities, identifying support for the two young carers and exploring alternative ways of managing her anxiety.

The community support worker identified voluntary work as an area of interest for Julie, and together they spent time approaching suitable agencies. Julie was successful in her application as a volunteer and began working in the community. The young people in the family were offered support from a young carers support service, which they accepted. Because of the growing confidence between Julie and her community support worker (CSW), the former admitted her problems with debt, which she hadn't mentioned to other members of the team. The CSW assisted with negotiating issues around the Court summons and repayment. Citizens' advice was contacted and a meeting with a debt counsellor arranged. The CSW assisted Julie in contacting all the companies to whom she owed money (while waiting for the CAB appointment) and supported her in visits to the Benefits Agency and the County Court.

With the input of the CSW, Julie felt confident enough to liaise with the District Council (Housing issues) and the Water/Gas/Electricity suppliers (arrears).

After some months, Julie negotiated her own increase to her voluntary hours and applied for a placement relating to vocational training. Julie now feels confident enough to fully engage with all aspects of self-management in the home and in the community. Further self-harming and hospital admissions have so far been avoided.

engaged in activities to help others while also receiving support themselves.

5. *Therapeutic supports.*

One of the most frequent everyday sayings is: 'there must be a cure for this'. One of the myths of modern life is that there must be some form of 'magic bullet' to deal with every health situation. So on one side there is a pull towards medication as a supposedly quick cure, and on the other there is a push against from publicised examples of medical interventions going wrong.

The power of the drugs companies is also an issue and recently Support Coalition International, the United States survivor rights organisation, has accused the makers of '*A Beautiful Mind*', the film about the Nobel prize winning mathematician, John Nash, and his struggle with a schizophrenic illness, of deliberately subverting Nash's message that he controlled his symptoms and rebuilt his life without medication, to an end line where he is stating that he is taking the newer form of antipsychotics (Kate Somerside, 'A Beautiful Spin', *Mental Health Today*, May 2002).

The Sainsbury Centre's User Perspectives report, (Rose, 2001) demonstrates that 'Users do not show a blanket rejection, or a blanket acceptance of their medication. In a user-focused interview, they discriminate between different questions and show that they balance the cost and the benefits of being on psychotropic medication' (p53).

The Mental Health Foundation's study shows a very similar finding:

One of the key things to emerge from a reading of interviews on the subject of medication is that of ambivalence. Many people have very mixed feelings about taking medication whether or not they found it helpful. It carried with it associations of long-term illness, concerns about physical health and potential long-term damage, particularly where side-effects were found distressing.

Mental Health Foundation,
November 1999: p37.

Diana Rose, for the Sainsbury Centre, points out that there is a huge significance in the way that general practitioners and psychiatrists are prepared to negotiate medication levels with their patients. Those who felt they still had some control over what they were prescribed had a greater sense of overall control of their lives. As we have seen from the Westminster Study, medication itself is very much only part of a strategy within a wider perspective of

Figure 11: The seven principles in relationship (Biestek, 1976).

First Direction: The *need* of the client	Second Direction: The *response* of the caseworker	Third Direction: The *awareness* of the client	The name of the *principle*
1 To be treated as an individual			1 Individualisation
2 To expresss feeings		The client is somehow *aware* of the caseworker's sensitivity, understanding, and response	2 Purposeful expression of feelings
3 To get sympathetic response to problems	The caseworker is *sensitive* to, *understands*, and appropriately *responds* to these needs		3 Controlled emotional involvement
4 To be recognised as a person of worth			4 Acceptance
5 Not to be judged			5 Nonjudgemental attitude
6 To make his own choices and decisions			6 Client self-determination
7 To keep secrets about self			7 Confidentiality

environmental and social supports strategies and services.

When I experienced my own bout of depressive illness, two of the things that impressed me most about my GP was firstly her very human reaction to the condition I was in, and her anger at the state in which I arrived in her surgery and her view of the circumstances which had led to my illness. Also the clear descriptions she gave me of the medication she felt would be most appropriate, and giving me a great deal of control as to when to start it. To be honest, my advice as a professional and as a friend to someone in my situation would have been something along the lines of that it was very much their choice, but that medication could be a very helpful aid in becoming strong enough to bring other strategies into play to recover one's health. In practice, however, I was very wary about taking medication for all the reasons outlined in the user surveys: I didn't want to lose control, I was worried about side effects, I wanted to do it all myself, and even relatively small things troubled me, for instance I was running the London Marathon for my local MIND as part of my recovery strategy, and feared that anti-depressants would cause me a dry mouth – very difficult for marathon running! In hindsight, I should have taken my GP's advice to start the anti-depressants earlier than I did, but her willingness to allow me maximum control, while keeping an eye on my condition, was very helpful for my sense of autonomy.

6. *Professional support.*

Fundamental to the relations with professionals was a person-centred approach which accorded people a sense of respect, dignity, value, equality and being heard. As described above, I found a human reaction, rather than professional detachment, to be extremely helpful, and this is one of the major challenges for professionals in being warm and genuine, yet keeping that emotional involvement detached enough to not disempower the person one is working with, and to ensure that professional knowledge is brought into play. These values were well defined in the work of Felix Biestek in the 1960s and 1970s in his classic text: *The Casework Relationship*, Biestek, 1976.

Work on values in social and health care have understandably developed since the 1970s; especially around issues of empowerment, but the kind of values and attitudes desired by users in the various studies (Rose, 2001, Mental Health Foundation, 1999, Macdonald and Sheldon, 1997) demonstrate the same concerns around:

• being valued
• genuineness
• accessibility
• continuity
• help to maintain and regain independence

Strategies for Living states that 'The most helpful professional interventions combined both emotional and practical support; people tended to experience such workers as genuinely interested and caring' (p44). These were precisely the kind of values and behaviours found useful by users and carers in the Leeds Survey (Leeds, 1997) 'I find my social worker excellent, reliable, reassuring, punctual, helpful and genuine'. (service user). 'It's good to be able to talk to a person who understands my son's problems'. (carer).

As society becomes considerably more complicated, supporting existing networks, where appropriate, and reinforcing individuals and groups' coping strategies, becomes ever more vital. This is particularly important in issues around culture and race where it's all too easy to cut across existing mechanisms for support.

> ... (the social workers) help me fill out all the forms and go to the right people to speak to about getting a place of my own ... and how to deal with it and learning how to pay my rent and how to manage my money, and how to buy clothes and shopping and stuff like that. They teach you all those kinds of things, of basically how to live independently, they teach you, and it's been a great help. Because without that support, I wouldn't have been able to have made it.
> service user quoted in *Mental Health Foundation*,
> November 1999.

7. Talking therapies and complementary therapies.

There is a danger that we see talking therapies and complementary therapies as a middle class occupation. In fact, both of these go back to primary needs to talk, to be listened to, to have thoughts and feelings reflected back to one, to retain control of one's coping and healing strategies, to seek for a reduction in stress and a better harmony between mind and body.

I am concerned that some people I meet in long-term therapy have gained a form of personalised insight but at the expense of an ability to relate to other people.

There is some evidence that these therapies are less available to people from black and ethnic minorities and those from more deprived socio-economic groups. Again, the issue of race and culture is most important:

> ... You tend to feel more at home with a black person ... it is just a general feeling, you feel more relaxed and you can talk, you can be more open with yourself talking with a black person rather than talking with a white person ...
> Afro-Caribbean man.

> ... When I came I wanted to talk to somebody of my own culture and my own age and they have children

and problems, and they should, suppose to understand what I'm going through.
> Asian woman.

Assumptions are, however, extremely dangerous. Increasingly, people do not feel themselves to be in one culture, but perhaps moving from one culture to another, or part of inter-cultural, multi-cultural groupings, so in all other aspects of mental health, the key worker needs to explore carefully with the user how they see their needs. (See Fernando, 1995.)

8. Personal and self-help strategies.

As Thompson writes in *Existentialism and Social Work*:

> Discovering that one is responsible for one's own actions can be a very disturbing and destabilising realisation, but it is also a moment of liberation – a liberation for the illusions which deny freedom. As such, it is a significant source of potential empowerment.
> Thompson, 1992.

In the end, however helpful our family, friends and professionals are, we are as a service user, a carer, a professional, or an amalgam of all of these, essentially alone with our own history, strengths and weaknesses, belief systems etc.

Some of the self-help strategies described in the literature are:

- positive self-help approaches
- managing distress and negotiating peace
- sport and physical exercise
- approaches to physical health
- relaxation and stress relief
- motivational approaches
- creativity
- spiritual and religious beliefs
- support of others

Fundamentally, there is another major connection between users, carers and professionals in that we all need to feel that there is a meaning and purpose to life in general and our life in particular. Without that, it is very difficult to face the daily grind.

A recognition of the spiritual dimension of everybody is essential (see NSF, September 2001, Health Education Authority, 1999; Copsey, 1997; Copsey, 2001; Mental Health Foundation, 1997):

- Spirituality is all about making sense of our lives and discovering meaning and purpose.
- A belief in a personal God or gods or a specific belief system, may be individual or based within a faith community.

Case Example 5

Give me my life back

How a man diagnosed with schizophrenia can be helped out of his apathy.

Case study

The names of all service users mentioned have been changed.

Situation: Roger Castlemaine is a 48-year-old white male who has been a diagnosed schizophrenic since he was 18-years-old. He receives depot injections for his condition. Castlemaine, whose son is likewise on medication, also looks after his 82-year-old mother.

Problem: Castlemaine feels that his life has been wasted, although he has been grateful to hold down the occasional low-paid job. He believes very strongly that his injections have made him 'a pathetic man'. He feels so 'un-alive' while on medication (he uses Largactil, an anti-psychotic drug) that music, once a passionate love, now does nothing to lift him. He feels he has no emotions – he can't get happy, sad or angry. He has been told that this is his schizophrenia but he rejects that. He believes he is suffering from drug-induced apathy. He says he would rather be ill than be on medication. Feeling so numb and 'out of it' has depressed him, to such an extent that he has even considered suicide. During these low points, Castlemaine has embraced Christianity, finding a comfort and understanding, he says, that has not been on offer to him from his doctors. His son takes olanzapine which, says Castlemaine, helps him to cope 'without turning him into a zombie'. His 30 years of medication have, for Castlemaine, quite simply 'ruined my life'.

Mark Trewin, approved social worker, Bradford District Care Trust

Roger Castlemaine's situation is a reminder to mental health professionals that service users have to consider the effects of the medication that they take against the possible benefits. While medication can help, the side-effects mean that there are also major risks involved. Mental health professionals are increasingly discussing these issues with service users and supporting them to find a balance. An attitude of 'compliance at any cost' can be damaging.

In this situation, Castlemaine would probably benefit from a fresh assessment of his health and social needs. The needs of people with a stable but long-term mental health problem can often be overlooked. It appears that there are many issues that are important to Castlemaine in addition to medication, such as his role as carer, his physical health, his spiritual needs, his access to employment and leisure activities. This assessment should be undertaken from his point of view and with his full involvement and should lead to a care plan that identifies the changes he feels are important and how these would be achieved. Castlemaine is likely to gain a great deal from feeling much more involved with the way his care is planned and carried out.

The mental health team could support Castlemaine to change or reduce his medication in an attempt to reduce the side-effects. There may be alternative ways of supporting his positive mental health. It could be time to review the relevance of his diagnosis. It is important that he feels that he is being listened to and this may be a vital part of that process.

His role as a carer, both for his mother and son, should be tackled, as he may need support in this area that is separate to his own mental health needs. Castlemaine is depressed and has expressed suicidal thoughts. Giving him the opportunity to express how he feels, while attempting to resolve some of the issues could reduce the risk of increased depression.

The important principle in this case is that people with a mental health problem have a right to live full and satisfying lives. If our treatment of mental health problems compromises this basic right then we need to reconsider the way that we support people.

Gill Rowe-Aslam, team leader, Bradford home treatment service, Bradford District Care Trust.

Roger Castlemaine's aspirations have not been fulfilled. He gives a clear impression that, despite his achievements, he wishes for more. He does not feel motivated enough to actively pursue his interests. In addition to this he describes his emotions as very flat, which appears to be a source of further frustration to him.

This hinders his ability to care for himself, has a negative impact on his self-esteem and prevents him from feeling able to offer any practical or emotional support to his son or mother.

Through the care programme approach the issue of a medication review could be addressed in a structured and focused way. Castlemaine may wish to explore alternative types of medication or treatment. The benefits of complementary medicine and alternative approaches could be also be considered. For example, the Hearing Voices Network – a self-help organisation for people, many of whom have been diagnosed as schizophrenic, or the Hearing Voices workbook[1] (a way of understanding and managing voices). He may also wish to be involved in a local user or self-help organisation, which he may use for support of his own needs, or prefer to be more actively involved in supporting others. It may be helpful for an advocate to accompany him to a meeting to assist him in representing his views.

Assuming the outcome of this was successful, Castlemaine would hopefully feel more in control and motivated. This would then give him and his care co-ordinator room to address the further issues of his daily activities and pursuing interests. He could be supported in taking up job-related training with a view to re-entering employment.

If Castlemaine has found Christianity, a source of comfort and understanding for him, it is important for this to be acknowledged and any wishes to work within a spiritual framework should also be explored.

It appears that Castlemaine actually holds two roles in all this, in that he is both the cared for and the carer. Therefore, not only is he entitled to an assessment of his own needs, but also of any additional needs he may have as a carer of both his son and 82-year-old mother.

[1]J Downs (ed), *Coping with Voices and Visions*, Hearing Voices Network. Available from 91 Oldham Street, Manchester M4 1LW. Tel/fax: 0161 834 5768.

User view

I find this man's situation tragic, writes Kay Sheldon. There are many people with long-standing mental health problems who have been overlooked by current mental health practice and policy. It is often easier to 'maintain' us, carrying on with the same regime, year after year, without considering the impact this has on quality of life.

Roger's mental health needs should be completely reviewed by his community mental health team in a user-centred and holistic way, including a review of his medication. In addition, his social set-up and his occupational status should be discussed in depth with him. The team should establish a mutually respectful partnership with Roger, encouraging and supporting him to make decisions himself.

I have little doubt that, having been there myself, Roger's apathy is due to his medication. It may be that Roger would like to come off medication altogether – this should be supported and facilitated by the team, including developing a contingency plan with Roger, should he start to become unwell. A different anti-psychotic, maybe one of the newer ones, or an anti-depressant or both may be preferable alternatives to Roger. He could find it quite difficult to come off his current medication because of withdrawal reactions, especially from the Largactil, which, contrary to popular belief does cause such effects. Also, psychologically it can be daunting to let go of something that has been part of your life for so long. Whatever is decided, it is important that Roger feels both in control of his mental health and supported enough to take this responsibility.

At 48, Roger obviously feels that he has missed out on a large slice of life. Counselling may be helpful in coming to terms with his loss and to help him think more positively about his future. Counselling may also be beneficial when, or if, Roger recovers his emotions, which can be difficult to cope with after such a long time of numbness.

On a practical level, Roger could be helped to make changes to his life and to rekindle some of his former passions. Help with caring for his mother might be useful, if he is tied to the home. Efforts could be made to reignite his musical interests.

Voluntary work or doing a course could help him put some meaning back into his life. Roger deserves all the help the services can offer him to move on from just existing to actually living once again.

Kay Sheldon is a mental health service user.

Reprinted by kind permission of *Community Care*, 9–15 May, 2002.

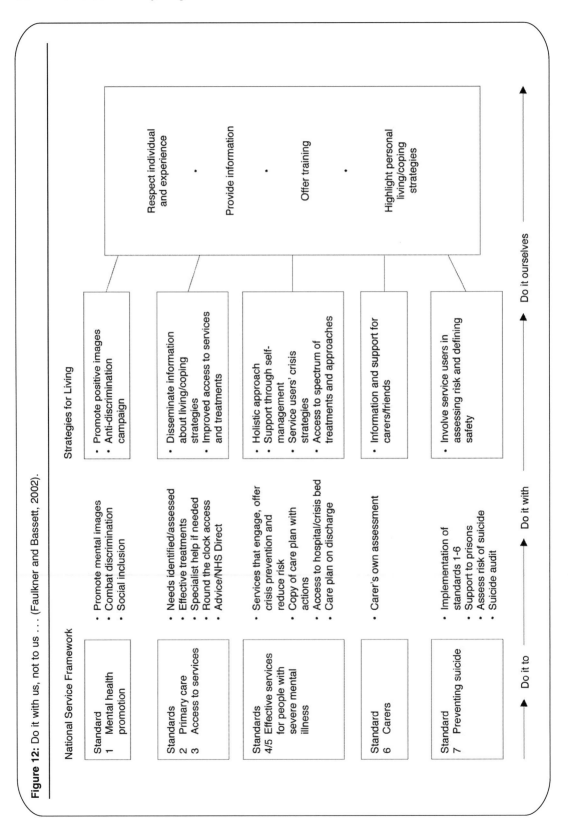

Figure 12: Do it with us, not to us . . . (Faulkner and Bassett, 2002).

- Faith communities may have very different approaches to mental distress and mental illness – either supportive and nurturing or negative and excluding.

John Swinton's work on *Spirituality and Mental Health Care* states that: 'Systematic reviews of the literature have consistently reported that aspects of religious and spiritual involvement are associated with desirable mental health outcomes' (Swinton, 2001: p68), though clearly there can be negative aspects as well. The long-standing faith communities need to be less defensive about the broader aspects of spirituality, while mental health professionals need to listen to what users are saying about the spiritual aspects of their lives.

   9. *Making sense.*

When I was Director of Operations for Staffordshire Social Services, I worked closely with partners on developing a mental health strategy for the North of the county. Some very participatory workshops elicited a strategic direction which made sense to all partners, and had some very vivid and powerful depictions of the sort of services that users and carers would find helpful. 18 months on, the vivid imagery had been 'professionalised' out of the strategy, and I couldn't recognise any of the issues that users had raised in the ways that they had described them!

In work on a one-to-one basis, with groups and communities, the language and the concepts have to be such that they make sense to everybody and are owned by everybody. In terms of the National Service Framework, an approach that many other parts of health and social care many other countries are wanting to copy, it is worth looking at this also from a user's point of view. Figure 12 by Alison Falkner and Thurstine Bassett brings a user perspective and language to the process.

   10. *Making connections.*

Frameworks such as the NSF aim to bring together what users and carers want from services and how national policy envisages the delivery of Mental Health Services. **Effective social work has to be about bridging the overarching strategy with the individual aspirations of people.**

I was struck the other day by a mental health manager with over 20 years experience in social services relating to me 'what got her out of bed' every morning even when the pressures of work were intolerable:

> *When I joined the social work staff at XXXXXXX hospital, I met early on 'Glynis' who had been compulsorily admitted to XXXXXXXX in her early twenties as a 'moral defective' because she'd had an illegitimate child. 'Glynis' certainly wasn't suffering from a mental illness, and wouldn't have gone within a million miles of the hospital in today's climate. My greatest satisfaction was being able to place Glynis, now in her early seventies, in a community setting of her choice, with other friends; and the spur to my continued commitment to social work is helping people to try and take control of their lives and supporting people who without help would be denied the life experiences which we all wish for ourselves.*
>
> senior manager, Mental Health Services (social work background, but managing health and social care services).

Professionals and managers have a tendency to overlay user and carer issues – usually expressed in powerful and compelling images – with a coating of jargon. Faulkner and Bassett's diagram is extremely useful because it translates the language of strategy into the lived and living experience of people who use (and may in the future require) services.

We use the words 'modernise' in the health and social care world, and so we should, but we also work in a post modern world where the 'grand narratives' of the past have lost some of their force, and we need to listen to 'the view from below and within, individual narratives, different viewpoints, the personal experience' (Professor Anthony Clare, in the foreword to Priebe, S. and Slade, M., 2002, *Evidence in Mental Health Care.* Hove, Brunner-Routledge).

At the end of the day, services are for those who use them, not for those who provide them.

Chapter 5

The Skilled Helper – The Role of the Social Worker

I am very satisfied with my social worker; she is very helpful and always treats me with the utmost respect.
Quoted in SSI Inspection, September 2001.

Social work can make a particularly valuable contribution to improving the quality and delivery of services, given that the causes and consequences of poor mental health are significantly influenced by the environment of which we are all a part. Social work is by nature holistic in approach and views the individual within a wider context of their personal, familial, cultural and socio-economic circumstances. Its ethos is on empowerment and promoting independence through a focus on 'working with' rather than 'doing to' which helps to increase personal achievement, self-fulfilment and create a much stronger sense of citizenship.
David Joannides, Director of Social Services and Chair of the ADSS Mental Health Strategy Group.

The social worker is the point of contact at a time of crisis or focused need. They have a professionalism that offers a useful distance from the problem in hand and allows them to deal dispassionately with the situation . . . The person who becomes a social worker wants to make a difference to the lives of people and communities, and their commitment is often clear to see in their practice. The practice of social work can be frustrating due to lack of suitable resources. Social workers should be closely involved in planning services for people and communities as they are best placed to provide advice and ideas on the needs, gaps and processes of communities and disadvantaged groups.
co-ordinator of a voluntary sector service.

A lot has been written recently, in Community Care and elsewhere, about the extent to which social workers are undervalued. But in Mental Health work their value is beyond doubt.
Margaret Clayton, Chairperson of the Mental Health Act Commission, *Community Care*, 23rd May, 2002: p38–9.

Social work is a very practical job; it is about protecting people and changing their lives.
Jacqui Smith, MP, Health Minister, 22nd May 2002, announcing the details of the new curriculum for the Social Work Degree Course.

Placing yourself where the user is

At a particularly hectic time as a director of social services, I contracted a bad sinus infection. Wanting to get back to full health as soon as possible, I queued up for evening surgery and was seen by a GP in his 50s who, when I said what work I was in, launched into a eulogy about the practice-based social worker (and yes, I did contact the social worker and her manager the next day to give them the positive feedback). What were the most important factors in her work, I asked the GP?

> *She seems to be able to put herself where the patient (sic) is and, as somebody who has been in general practice many years, the life we live now seems to me to be a lot more complicated than it used to be; the social worker can find her way through the maze which is society today in a way that makes things easier for the patient and for us.*

It has always struck me from the time I was a social work trainee on attachment to a GP surgery in the mid 1970s that there is, or should be, a natural affinity between social workers and general practitioners. Both have to pull off the conjuring trick of working with individuals, with their unique natures and circumstances, and help them cope with and develop in an increasingly complex world, where people cannot depend on the certainties they once put their trust in.

As a generic (general) social worker in the late 1970s/early 1980s, I worked with an older, single mother, with a very poor self image, who had married late in life, given birth to a daughter, and then faced the tragedy of her husband dying suddenly. Mrs 'T' found herself not only grieving but **extremely** angry with life for snatching happiness away from her, and angry with her daughter, that it was her daughter who was still alive and not her husband.

This was a very middle class family and although it soon became clear to the GP and her neighbours that 'Sally', the daughter, was at risk, and that Mrs 'T' was in acute mental distress, nobody had felt it appropriate to contact social services, because middle class families in middle class neighbourhoods coped – didn't they?! As Mrs T's mental health deteriorated, however, her expressions of pain became more extreme, and her attitude towards 'Sally' declined. Neighbours ran out of capacity to cope with the demands and the anxiety.

When social services were eventually involved, Mrs T was very frank about her feelings of extreme anger to her daughter, and the occasional desire, especially when washing her hair in the bath, to actually drown her. A psychiatrist and clinical psychologist were involved, but the day-to-day work was through a social worker and a family support worker. The social history was especially vital to the psychiatrist and GP, as it was through this that Mrs T's deep-rooted sense of worthlessness and that life had 'cheated' her became starkly evident. The intensive work by the social worker and family support worker was required to ensure both the safety of Sally in the short term, but also the viability of the family unit in the long run. If the professionals had completely taken control of the situation, then Mrs T's feelings of worthlessness would have been reinforced: 'I'm a worthless wife who couldn't save her husband from the heart attack that killed him; I'm a worthless mother because you've taken my child away'.

Some excellent work was done by the psychologist, but as Mrs T's self-awareness and recognition of the issues troubling her surfaced, the danger to 'Sally' increased as the mother became more volatile. The psychologist was not aware of this, but the social worker and family support worker were. It became clear that therapeutic work to heal Mrs T's wounds could not be carried any further until Sally was more comprehensively safeguarded. Mrs T was persuaded to request Sally's reception into care in a partnership arrangement with the Local Authority, and she was informally admitted to the local psychiatric hospital under the 1959 Mental Health Act. She was treated for depression and therapeutic work undertaken to address her feelings of low self-worth. The social worker continued to work with Mrs T and supported Sally in the foster home. Sally was a very intelligent and strong-minded nine-year-old who was quite aware of the danger she had been in while in her mother's care and the ambivalent feelings her mother had for her. Despite this, she was very clear that she wished to return to her mother as soon as possible, and this was expressed with some hostility towards the social worker.

In the end, Mrs T came out of hospital with her depression lifted, and a number of feelings about herself and her circumstances ameliorated if not fully resolved. Sally was considered to be no longer at immediate risk, and she was very clear that she wished to return home. Intensive work continued from the social worker, and

even more especially by the family support worker who worked with Mrs T on the care tasks with Sally which Mrs T found particularly difficult. The social worker co-ordinated input with health staff and rebuilt the capacity for support within the local community, through the church that Mrs T and Sally belonged to. In the end, the family and the community learned to cope again.

For the social worker, there was the challenge of assisting a parent and child to rebuild a relationship both in the present and for the future; high risk elements around childcare and mental health; the need to balance the safety of the child which was paramount with the fact that any increasing feeling of powerlessness and worthlessness on Mrs T's part would have made the mother-child relationship non-viable in the future; there was complex networking to take place both with health professionals, with communication between the GP and the consultant psychiatrist, not always of the first order, and competing agendas between a concentration by the Mental Health professionals on the mother, and the social worker and GP balancing need to concentrate on the safety of the child as well; there was the imperative for the social worker to supervise the family support worker, without whose character and skills the child would have been at risk and the relationship might not have been viable in the long run.

Without social work intervention, the child would not have been protected adequately and the mother-child relationship would almost certainly have broken down permanently. The social worker's balancing of risk around the paramount safety of the child but also her long-term need for a stable relationship with her mother; the need to network with professional bodies and the wider community; knowledge of child care and mental health law; an understanding of psychological processes for both the child and the mother; and holding both the short-term and the long-term issues together creates a pressure on the social worker which not many professionals would wish to have.

Professor Andrew Cooper, of the Tavistock, in a recent article, quotes a friend and colleague as saying:

'I don't think they really understand in Health what we mean when we call ourselves a therapeutic service. It is not about individual treatment programmes, it is about all the things that you and I have talked about over the

years – a total response to the complex dynamics of family plus professional system that you get presented with'.

Cooper, March 2002: p7.

As we have seen from the preceding chapters, users value:

- Somebody to work alongside them as they make sense of themselves and themselves within the world around them.
- Being valued as individuals and as citizens.
- Help with both the emotional and the practical side of life.
- Assistance in working through the maze of agencies.
- Mediation in both family, group and community relationships.
- Balancing personal liberty with care.

Carers' value:

- Appreciation of their individuality and citizenship.
- Help in preserving their essential relationship with the person cared for as husband/wife, mother/father, son/daughter, rather than being viewed primarily as a 'carer'.
- Accurate and accessible information.
- Assistance in finding their way through the maze of agencies, benefits etc.
- Contact with other carers with similar circumstances.
- Time to talk with an empathetic listener about the particular pressures on them as carers, and their aspirations for the future.

Both users and carers wish to be able to influence service policy and systems in a dynamic way (see Beresford, June, 2002).

Societies and governments have expectations as well. Whether we define government in the highly optimistic tones of Charles James Fox:

What is the end of all government? Certainly the happiness of the governed.

Charles James Fox, MP, House of Commons,
1st December 1783.

Or, in the words of the French proponent of minimal government:

To be governed is to be inspected, spied upon, directed, law-driven, regulated, preached at, controlled, censored . . .

Pierre-Joseph Proudhon.

Or again, the pragmatic, utilitarian approach which informs much of modern governance:

That action is best which procures the greatest happiness for the greatest numbers.

The words of Francis Hutcheson, developed
by Bentham and John Stuart Mill.

As Banks, Davies and others point out:

Social workers are not autonomous professionals whose guiding ethical principles are solely about respecting and promoting the self-determination of service users. They are employed by agencies, work within the constraints of legal and procedural rules and must also work to promote the public good or the well-being of society in general.

Banks, 1995: p31.

And Davies:

*The practice of social work takes place almost wholly as a result of **either** statutory legislation or policy decisions taken by politicians in central or local government. The functions of the social worker and the focus of her work are not self-selected but are politically sanctioned and authorised by the agent which employed her. The point that makes as many questions as it answers, but it does at least indicate the source of social work legitimacy, and emphasises that social workers are not, and can never be, a law unto themselves.*

Davies, 1994 (See also Smale, et al., 2000: Ch. 1).

Governments therefore desire:

- The fulfilment of social objectives through the carrying out of legislation and agency practice.
- The promotion of citizenship and the healthy functioning of individuals, families and communities.
- The maintenance of equilibrium between the liberty of the subject and the safety of the subject and other people.

Of course, as we can see from the case description given above of Mrs T and Sally, there are numerous tensions inherent in the effective delivery of social work. Users and carers are often lumped together in policy documents and statements, and yet their needs are often different and there may well be confliction. The state and its legislation may be beneficent, but can also be oppressive. Britain's uneasy compromise between American libertarianism and European communitarianism is under pressure from both sides. We tend to regard 'the Law' as neutral, but it is a reflection of society, especially as Mental Health law has oscillated between care, legalism, treatment, rights and safety. There are considerable debates now both within and without the legal profession as to whom the current legislative framework serves, with the police service for example being concerned about the balance between the rights of the victim and the rights of the alleged perpetrator. (See, for example, Neyroud and Beckley, 2001.) As Giovanni Battista Montini once remarked:

> *Legislation is necessary but is not sufficient for setting up true relationships of justice and equality ... If beyond legal rules there is no deeper feeling of respect for a service for others, then equality before the law can serve as an alibi for flagrant discrimination, continued exploitation and actual contempt.*
>
> Quoted in Philpot, 1986: p148.

It is into this complex and conflictual environment that social work has to operate. Not only are there obvious dichotomies between different individuals and groups but also within the world of the person one is working with. In such a world, the utilisation of precise science, the application of the scalpel and laser are not appropriate. In essence, the social worker is a skilful mariner, navigating a fragile bark among the shoals and reefs and currents of life together with those they are working with. As my social work tutor, Hugh England asserts:

> *The source of social work's potential strength, and the conviction of its proponents, is the very fact that it does not separate the world experienced by those in need of help into component elements. Such experience is always a complex, composite experience, it is always a unique synthesis; yet it cannot be impossible to construct such a synthesis, because the client – and everyone – does so all the time. The strength of the able worker lies in his [sic] ability accurately to join the client in a construction and experience of this synthesis. It is only through such sharing that people sometimes say to others . . .'you seem to understand' – and we know that to be understood by others is a necessary and a therapeutic experience.*
>
> England, 1986.

> *Nurses are not taught to manage conflict or be agents of social control. If they had wanted to do that role, I guess they would have trained to be social workers.*
>
> social worker in a multi-disciplinary team.

Historical roots and routes

> *... there seems something else in life besides time, something which may conveniently be called 'value', something which is measured not by minutes or hours, but by intensity, so that when we look at our past, it does not stretch back evenly but piles up into a few notable pinnacles, and when we look at the future it seems sometimes a wall, sometimes a cloud, sometimes a sun, but never a chronological chart.*
>
> Forster, *Aspects of the Novel*,
> The Clark Lecturers, 1927.

> *The unifying element . . . is the professional skill of the social worker whether deployed in field work, in primary care, in residential or day care, or in hospital.*
>
> Better Services for the Mentally Ill, 1975: p23.

As Jordan states:

> *In societies which are relatively simple in construction, there are no social workers. Vulnerable people 'are looked after within the extended family or the tribe. Unconventional behaviour is either tolerated, venerated or punished by retributive methods.*
>
> Jordan, 1984: p31.

Younghusband makes a similar point about social care being regarded 'as something private or as an attitude, a concern for welfare, rather than as a practice based upon knowledge and skill', (Younghusband, 1978: p24). This is not so different from how nursing was regarded in the mid 19th century, because, after all, anyone can nurse and the portrayal of the professional nurse, such as Mrs Gamp in Dickens's *Martin Chuzzlewit* (1843) is hardly flattering. The professionalism of the doctor also is not something which has been fixed for all time. The doctor in Flaubert's *Madame Bovary* or Mr Perry in Jane Austen's *Emma* have an ambiguous professional persona and before that the English radicals used to refer to the doctors' limited skills in 'purging and bleeding' (see Hill, 1975) in the same way that some users now refer to 'chemical straightjackets'.

As Midwinter points out (Midwinter, 1994) the mediaeval monasteries were the first welfare state, and the alms-houses were the forerunners of both the hospitals and care homes. When they were abolished at the Reformation, the state had to find other means to alleviate the direct effects of poverty and ill-health while ensuring that social unrest was averted.

The 1601 Elizabethan Poor Law set out a system of outdoor relief, reversed in 1834 by the new Poor Law and its emphasis on institutions.

Andrew Scull, Professor of Sociology at the University of California, highlights 'the transformations underlying the move towards institutionalisation' being tied 'to the growth of the capitalist market system and to its impact on economic and social relationships' (Scull, 1984: p24). Increasing geographical mobility (echoed in the 20th and 21st centuries); the alienation and anonymity of the urban slums; the destruction of the old paternal relationships; the breakdown of rural patterns as described in Hardy's *Far from the Madding Crowd*; and rapid technological progress (again an echo in our own day) meant that 'the situation of the poor and dependent classes became simultaneously more visible and more desperate' (Scull: p22).

Scull identifies a number of connected features to distinguish deviance and its control in modern society:

- The substantial involvement of the state, and the emergence of a highly rationalised and generally centrally administered and directed social control apparatus.
- The treatment of many types of deviance in institutions providing a large measure of segregation from the surrounding community.
- The careful differentiation of different sources of deviance, and the subsequent confinement of each variety to the ministration of 'experts', (Scull: p15).

This drive towards greater organisation would have been recognised by Edwin Chadwick as he pushed forward the social reforms of the mid Victorian era (see Midwinter, 1994: Chapter 4.) Though we are indebted to Chadwick in many ways for his social environmental reforms – in fact had Chadwick been able to enlist wider support among the governing classes, we might be living today in a country with a markedly cleaner environment and a health service less concentrated on individual pathology (see Small, 1998) – the Earl of Shaftesbury's concern for people in mental distress was much more based on principles of care, than Chadwick's preoccupation for social order.

The historical pendulum described in Chapter 2 is in full flow in mental health services from the mid 19th century.

For those at the receiving end of care, treatment, control etc., the picture could be very stark and there is nobody like Charles Dickens to describe the social environment and our need to work towards a common good so as to avoid it 'raining social retributions' (*Dombey and Son*, 1846) and the reaction of those who were deprived to the power of the state on the one hand and the machinations of an unregulated private sector, e.g. Dotheboys Hall (*Nicholas Nickleby*, 1838) on the other.

Dickens's description of Betty Higden in *Our Mutual Friend* (1864) she of 'indomitable purpose and a strong constitution', is demonstrative of the poor's attitude to the state:

God help me and the like of me! – how the worn-out people that do come down to that, get driven from post to pillar and pillar to post, a-purpose to tire them out! Do I never read how they are put off, put off – how they are grudged, grudged, grudged, the shelter, or the doctor, or the drop of physic, or the drop of bread . . . then I say, I hope I can die as well as another, and I'll die without that disgrace (of entering the workhouse) . . . sooner than fall into the hands of those cruel jacks we read of, that dodge and drive, and worry and weary, and scorn and shame the decent poor.
Dickens, 1864, 1988 edition: p248.

It is Mrs Pardiggle, the visitor of the poor, with her certainties (*Bleak House*, 1853) who might be seen as the negative caricature of the social worker, whereas Esther Summerson , with her greater self-awareness could be speaking as a social work student when she says:

That I was inexperienced in the art of adapting my mind to minds very differently situated, and addressing them from suitable points of view. That I had not that delicate knowledge of the heart that must be essential to such a work. That I had much to learn, myself, before I could teach others and that I could not confide in my good intentions alone . . .
Bleak House, 1852, 1911 edition: p127.

As Bill Jordan points out in his admirable *Invitation to Social Work* (Jordan, 1984) it was the social reformer, Octavia Hill, who talked about the defining quality of relationship between her and her helpers and the tenants as 'respectfulness', a phrase which chimes very much with modern social work values (see below).

Hill added that 'each man (sic) has had his own view of life and must be freed to fulfil it . . . In many ways he is a far better judge of it than we, as he has lived through himself what we have only seen', (Jordan, 1984, p37 and 41).

The social reform tradition; the growth of therapeutic approaches stemming mainly from the USA and a local government strand began to come together, with some aspects of collision as well as cohesion in the 1950s.

Mental health social work encapsulates some of the tensions which exist in social work as a whole, and came to a head in the 1982 *Barclay Report* which argued that:

'The personal social services must develop a close working partnership with citizens focusing more closely on the community and its strengths' (p199), while the minority report by Robert Pinker stressed a more professional and casework approach (Pinker, 1982). The more highly qualified psychiatric social workers tended to be more readily found in the main psychiatric hospitals, while the mental welfare

Figure 13: Routes towards the social worker in mental health.

- 19th century social philanthropists:
  - social action
  - community approach
  - insistence on independence and self-help.
- American psychotherapy:
  - therapeutic approaches
  - understanding of history to unlock the present
  - advent of psychiatric social workers
- Local Government (Poor Law and afterwards):
  - social control
  - alleviation of extreme poverty
  - work with individuals and families
  - duly authorised officers and mental welfare officers

(See Timms, 1964; Jones, 1972, 1988; Younghusband, 1978; Butler and Pritchard, 1983; Olsen, 1984; Ulas and Connor, 2000; Heimler, 1967.)

officers came from the administrative and supervisory tradition within local authorities stemming from the Mental Health and Mental Treatment Acts of the early part of the 20th century. While Goldberg's studies in the early 1960s concluded that: 'Some understanding of the whole family constellation is essential before any plan for treatment can be formulated' (quoted in Younghusband, 1978: p167). Clearly much of the social work resource was in the wrong area to effect change.

Gradually, PSWs and mental welfare officers moved closer together. The Macintosh Report (1951) and the Younghusband Report (1959) both recommended extensive initiatives on training for social workers in mental health, and the 1968 Seebohm Report reinforced the value of social work for people experiencing mental ill-health:

The families of mentally disordered people tend to suffer from inter-related social disabilities which are often caused or aggravated by the mental disorder, which

---

Submission to the Department of Health from the Northamptonshire Approved Social Workers Standards Group on Proposed Reforms of the Mental Health Act, 1983

Historical Context

The first documented appointment of a trained mental health social worker in Britain was in 1928. From this inception, work was multi-disciplinary and provided new opportunities in ways of working with people with mental distress both within institutional and community setting. The role of the social worker was new and different from the profession of psychiatry which dominated hospitals at the time, and one of the tasks of the social worker encompassed recording service users' social history as part of their treatment plan.

In addition, social workers arranged after care services for patients being discharged. The underlying belief was that some did not need to be detained in hospital provided that adequate support services were available on discharge. Social workers at the time were the only mental health professionals to work across the hospital/community boundary.

In 1939, the Association of Psychiatric Social Workers turned down the BMA proposal that social workers should be registered as medical auxiliaries. At the time it was clear that the value base and theoretical orientation of social workers differed significantly from a medical model.

Despite this, the disciplines, at least locally, worked well together. The Social Work Department at St Crispin's Hospital, Northampton, in 1950, was described as being of 'great value in the total treatment effort', and in 1958, 'special attention was paid to outpatients and long-stay patients who wished to return to life outside the hospital'.

Mental health social workers were the first discipline to move out of psychiatric hospitals and base their practice within a community setting. They were also keen advocates of the closure of psychiatric hospitals, believing that, where possible, community resources should be mobilised to enable service users to have the opportunity to receive care and treatment outside institutions.

Social workers, therefore, have traditionally been, and continue to be concerned, with enabling people to have control over their lives, promoting people's right of citizenship and protecting those who are at risk in the least restricted way.

21st March 2000.

may precipitate breakdown or incapacitate the family for caring for the chronically sick member. The social worker should be concerned with the whole family, learning how to make a family diagnosis, and be able to take wide responsibility and mobilise a wide range of services.

Seebohm, 1968: para. 353.

Seebohm, of course, saw the creation of social services departments in 1971, bringing together the old children's, welfare and mental health departments, with children moving across from the Home Office, and mental health from the Health Service. This had the effect in some areas of simultaneously creating increased understanding of common issues across generations; effecting more 'clout' for social and community aspects of care; diluting some elements of specialist knowledge; dislocating some of the old relationships with other professionals and organisations in the mental health and learning disability fields.

The reintroduction of specialist social work, with a reasonable amount of permeability of experience and training between childcare, adult mental health and the mental health of old age, coupled with an acceptance, as Cooper points out, that one can have, and indeed should have, a foot in the two camps of social action and individual casework (Cooper, 2002: p8) has led to a strengthening of professional practice, coupled with a strong focus on the needs and rights of individual users and their families.

There is a danger that unless the values, knowledge and skills of social workers are not appreciated and nurtured, then the move into specialist mental health trusts could have the effect of emasculating the social and environmental perspectives, which are essential to counter the profound disadvantages in which many users with mental health needs find themselves.

Defining social work

Because social work performs so many different functions with such a range of individuals and groups, and interacts with a wide range of statutory and voluntary agencies, it is often difficult to define what it is in essence. As Hanvey and Philpot point out:

The problems social workers face are not so neatly dealt with as are problems faced by professionals who have to handle the arrest, the fire hose or the scalpel. The

material clues, the heartbeat and the pulse are, whatever the problems faced by others, more specific and scientific than what is often available to social workers.

Hanvey and Philpot, 1994: p3.

As Professor Thompson opines in his admirably clear *Understanding Social Work*, one can define social work in terms of theoretical constructs; through a descriptive approach and list of what social workers do; constructing it through an historical process; placing it in the broader context of social welfare; placing it in the tension between social stability and social change etc. (Thompson, 2000.)

Calling on his earlier work (Thompson, 1992) Thompson then considers an existential approach concentrating on:

- Ontology – concerning questions of human existence and meaning, and how existence presents us with a number of challenges that we have to meet and face in a variety of ways:
  - Life event challenges – those we face as we move from the cradle to the grave.
  - Challenges of circumstance and/or trauma confronting traumatic events and the issues we face as we try to reach our goals.
  - Socio-political challenges – stemming from our position in society, including poverty, racism, ageism, sexism, homophobia and other forms of exploitation.
- Uncertainty and flux – as we can see from all the case examples, appeal to a corpus of knowledge and personal experience is important, but 'a basic task for the social worker in very many situations is the management of uncertainty', (Thompson, 2000: p21) and one might add as well, the management of paradox.
- In these situations, social work practice needs to be:
  - Systematic – having a clear focus on what we are trying to achieve and why.
  - Reflective – reflecting on practice with an openness to change and develop (see also Brechin et al., 2000 and White and Taylor, 2000).
- Moral commitment – taking account of and attempting to ameliorate existing inequalities so that social work needs to be explicit about its value base and committed to demonstrating those values through 'supporting people in their struggles to break free from the disadvantage, discrimination and oppression they experience as a result of their social location' (Thompson, 2000: p23).

In trying to define social work, it might be interesting to look at some of the adverts recently published with backing from the Department of Health, ADSS and Local Government Association. The one featured here (Fig. 14) is of a young man, Patrick, who is isolated and in the midst of an episode of schizophrenia. Patrick's distress is featured, and the reasons for it, as well as behaviour stemming from his distress and the effect on his neighbours. The social worker is seen as addressing these issues in a practical way and interacting positively with the neighbours; what it doesn't show is an interpersonal response on an emotional level, and liaison with other professionals with whom Patrick clearly needs to be in contact. The advert states that:

'People can be fascinating, mystifying, rewarding. Social work is work with people, it's that simple and that complicated'.

The social work profession's own description of *The Social Work Task* is:

Social work is the purposeful and ethical application of personal skills in interpersonal relationships directed towards enhancing the personal and social functioning of an individual, family, group or neighbourhood.
BASW, 1977.

Most professions' descriptions of themselves have a certain pomposity about them, and some critics of social work rounded on this description of its task but, in effect, it's a pretty accurate summary of what social work does, though demographic, budgetary and policy pressures have tended to push social work away from having any impact on neighbourhoods in the way that it attempted to do in the 1970s and 1980s.

Social workers don't have the Benefit Agency's cash or the surgeon's scalpel (or laser); for them the instrument is the use of the self in situations where gauging where an individual is in the light of their mental and physical state, culture, past, beliefs, values, current circumstances etc., is immensely complex.

Individual social workers and the profession as a whole have to engage with the issues of care and control, especially in the context of the approved social worker (ASW) role (see Chapter 6) where the worker is accountable for their actions as an individual professional, rather than as a member of an agency.

Social workers derive their role from:

- The legislative framework.
- A policy framework.
- Its professional body.

- The agencies in which the workers operate, either statutory or voluntary.
- What users and carers need.

There are arguments as to the looseness or tightness of the task:

Those who commit themselves to social work contribute, in my view, to the sensitisation of our society. In doing so, they will not be popular; they must seek to hold, and to mediate in, the multiplicity of conflict in interpersonal relationships. They deal in shades of grey where the public looks for black and white. And they are bitterly resented for it. They are brokers in lesser evils, frequently faced with the need for choice followed by action whose outcome is unpredictable.
Professor Olive Stevenson, 1974, quoted in Hanvey and Philpot, 1994: p2.

'The truth is that social workers are employed to do a wide-ranging but quite specific job, which necessarily involves them in risk-taking, decision-making and the exercise of judgement' (Davies, *The Essential Social Worker*, quoted in Hanvey and Philpot, 1994: p3). There is also the argument as to how much social workers are agents of stability or change. Inevitably, if they are going to behave with integrity to the people they work with to serve, their colleagues, the agency they work for and their professional body (see Smale et al., 2000, and Thompson, 2000) they will look to reinforce those aspects of society which promote individual and social welfare (social stability) and seek to change negative and destructive aspects of society, such as discrimination (social change). Hugh England, in *Social Work as Art: Making Sense for Good Practice*, (England, 1986), quotes Noel and Rita Timms as saying 'Boundaries are loosely drawn and often permeable . . . this looseness constitutes one of the major challenges, if not one of the glories'. As England comments 'There is no doubt about the size of the challenge; I hope there will be no doubt that it is also a matter for glory' (p8).

The values of social work

They (the social workers) treat me with dignity and respect.
service user from the Westminster Study, 1997.

Social work values are directly at odds with the organisation that I am soon going to have to be employed by.
mental health social worker.

The love of liberty is the love of other people; the love of power is the love of ourselves.
William Hazlitt, 18th century essayist.

Case Example 6

T is a 44 year-old woman who has lived with severe mental illness for most of her adult life. Her first admission to hospital was at age 32, although she had been treated as an outpatient for the previous ten years. Her original diagnosis of depression began to move towards the more accurate diagnosis of schizophrenia over the years. By 1999, she had had 15 hospital admissions and had become a 'revolving door patient', with little hope, apparently destined to become a continuing care patient on a long stay ward.

Her husband, whom she met during her second hospital admission was an alcoholic and was usually in a very intoxicated state. Medical staff would not visit the home and would not listen to the couple's views. The home was in a severe squalid state; the carpets were soiled with faeces, most of the floor was covered in rubbish piled several feet in the room, cigarette butts were everywhere and opened tins of dog food were on every surface. The bed was soaked in urine and the smell permeated down to the ground floor of the block of flats, even though the flat was on the third floor and there were several doors between. T was incontinent, had congestive obstructive airway disease and mild cardiac failure. She smoked and drank (anything) constantly and had made numerous serious suicide attempts.

The medical staff was at a loss and requested help from social work staff who had only been invited to become involved at the point of compulsory detention. The nature of the request was more to do with keeping the alcoholic husband from visiting the ward and making demands on staff for his wife to go home. It was at this point that the social worker became involved and began the slow process of trying to gain the couple's trust to see what could be done.

It soon became very clear that the couple were very much in love and that despite their numerous difficulties, wanted to live together. It was from this premise that the social worker began the slow task of getting the couple to feel that they did have some power over the 'mighty medical system'. Through gentle encouragement, the couple were empowered, for the first time in their lives, to make some decisions about how they wanted to live and after a great deal of hard work, we were able to fund the fumigation, gutting and sterilisation of the flat, followed by re-decorating and furnishing it to a reasonable standard. The couple were involved throughout the entire process and although things did not run smoothly, we did not give up and the task was eventually completed. 'It would be fair to say that I experienced huge levels of resistance from medical staff, to the point where I almost gave up because of the pressure'.(SW)

A massive care package was organised to enable the couple to live in the flat. This included daily medication administration, cleaning, attention to personal hygiene, cooking, day-care and regular respite in a rehabilitation ward and becoming appointee for their financial benefits and organising payment of everything. The couple were again involved at each stage and slowly clear progress could be seen.

We are now 18 months on and the couple's lifestyle is unrecognisable. T has gained insight into her illness and is now able to talk about her own relapse symptoms. The flat is bright and clean. The care package has been reduced to only two hours each week and transport to attend a day centre. The couple shop and cook for themselves keep themselves clean and tidy and have, this week, taken back the total responsibility of their finances. Her husband's alcoholism is greatly improved and the couple have a quality of life that could never have been envisaged only a few years before.

The most difficulty was experienced in attempting to provide care on a flexible basis, with the local medical services being very rigid and unimaginative in their approach. Indeed, it is ironic that various medical establishments still complain, despite the exceptional progress that T has made.

Without social work intervention, T would be in a long stay ward, probably still very unwell, unhappy and unsafe and the couple would be apart. It is only the clear social work values that enabled this couple to have their current lifestyle and for T to be mentally stable and happy.

Figure 14: Advertisement for Social Work – 2002.

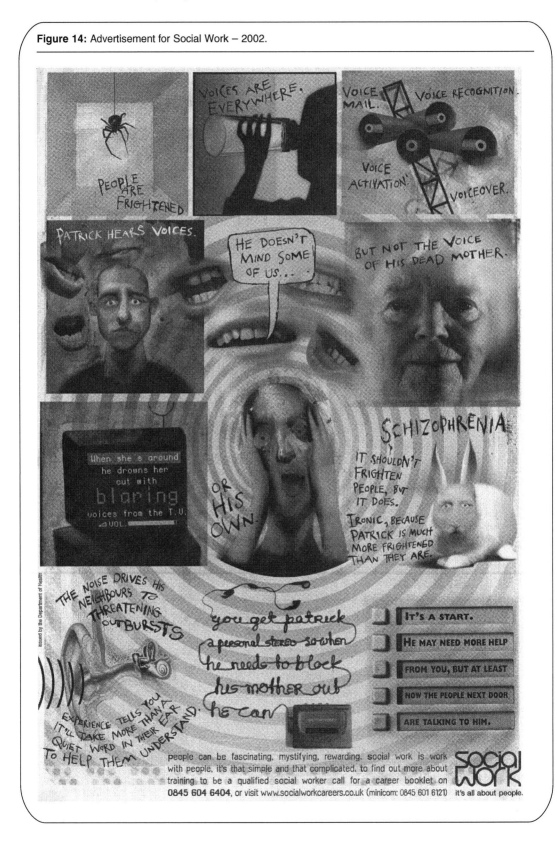

Only one thing prevailed – strength of character. Cleverness, creativeness, learning, all went down; only real goodness survived.

> Pierre d'Harcourt (Nazi concentration camp survivor) *The Real Enemy*, Longman, 1967.

As Zofia Butrym states in her *The Nature of Social Work*:

> *Implicit in the discussion of the nature of social work . . . is the fundamental importance of moral issues. This importance is derived from both the objectives of social work and the means by which it attempts to reach these objectives.*
>
> *Concern with the quality of human living which . . . is what social work is basically about, cannot operate in a moral vacuum but on the contrary must be based on certain beliefs. Regarding what constitutes 'a good life' and also on ethical considerations in relation to the ways by which such a good life can be sought and promoted.*
>
> Butrym, 1976: p40.

As Sarah Banks has flagged up in a book entirely devoted to ethics and values in social work (Banks, 1995: p4) ' "values" is one of those words that tends to be used rather vaguely and has a variety of different meanings'.

Dictionary definitions state that values are one's judgement of what is important in life, stemming from the Latin *valere*: to be strong, well, worth, and leading to the French *valoir*: to be worth, and related to the old Slavic *vlasti*: to govern. And indeed, it is essential to realise that as Professor Preston-Shoot so pertinently remarks 'Values are only as good as the actions they prompt', (Preston-Shoot, 1996: p31).

Ethics stems from the Greek *ethikos*: moral philosophy, and is the science of morals in human conduct; moral principles; rules of conduct. (See Thompson, 2000; Banks, 1995; Philpot, 1986; Butrym, 1976; Smale et al., 2000; Hanvey and Philpot, 1994; England, 1986; Davies, 1994; Braye and Preston-Shoot, 1995; British Association of Social Workers, 1986 and 2002).

Values have a vital role to play in organisations as long as they are 'real'. They:

- Provide the bedrock for the organisation – how people should behave to patients/clients/users/customers/partners, and towards each other.
- Creating a benchmark against which the prevailing culture and actions/responses of the organisation can be measured.
- Offering a framework for making sense of practice.

- Providing motivation and giving a sense to staff that they are valued and are adding value to the lives of others.

If values do not lead to appropriate actions, however, then they are, in that lovely North Midlands phrase: 'neither use nor ornament'! When I was Director of Operations for Staffordshire Social Services, two deaths of residents at the hospital for people with learning disabilities resulted in a team from Central Government being sent up, and led eventually to a county-wide partnership to close the hospital, re-provide the service and improve the lives of people with learning disabilities in the county. One of the deaths involved ward staff leaving a woman tied to a lavatory by her clothing while they went for lunch. The woman strangled herself in her efforts to get free. One of the Trade Union officials justified the event as the staff being under pressure and needing a break! The loss of dignity and freedom leading to the loss of the life of this woman happened not in Dickens 19th century, not even in the 1970s where a number of scandals led to a real drive to improve services and the values underpinning services, but in the mid 1990s!

I was recently concerned to hear of a consultant psychiatrist who questioned the use of 'citizens' as a description of users in the Statement of Principles and Practice produced by his trust. It seems to me that the tragedies where human beings are cruel to other human beings occur when we fail to recognise the shared humanity in the person facing us. That distancing, of course, comes so often from human kind's innate sense of separateness, dis-ease and anxiety, leading to a need to distance ourselves and see ourselves as superior.

Raymond Plant, summarising Immanuel Kant's philosophy in his book, *Social and Moral Theory in Casework*, says:

> *A man [sic] deserves respect as a potential moral agent in terms of his [sic] transcendental characteristic, not because of a particular conjunction of empirical qualities which he might possess. Traits of character might command admiration and other such responses, but respect is owed to a man, irrespective of what he does, because he is a man [sic].*
>
> see Plant, 1970, quoted in Philpot, 1986: p143 and Kant, *The Fundamental Principles of the Metaphysics of Ethics*, 1785.

Anti-oppressive practice is not an area which has a great deal of impact in Health Service thinking. It is

imperative that social workers continue to strive to achieve this, and challenge when it is not happening.
                                                           mental health social worker.

Of course, it is important that social work is not precious about the issue of the values. A whole range of professions who are concerned about the health, well-being and care of vulnerable people in the community e.g. youth workers, counsellors, clergy, chaplains, nurses, occupational therapists, housing officers etc., will subscribe to a broad set of values and professional identities, and some of the common themes will be commitment to:

- humanitarianism
- a value base
- a professional knowledge base
- a set of skills
- professional discretion and accountability
                                           Thompson, 2000: Ch. 1.

We have already come across the seven principles developed by Felix Biestek of Loyola University (Biestek, 1976: p17). These are still of great merit today, but as Banks makes clear, they were developed primarily within the context of voluntary, one-to-one casework relationship. Banks, Thompson and Braye and Preston-Shoot consider:

- The Kantian approach – with its accent on human beings as free individuals.
- Utilitarian approaches – where human beings are seen as free individuals, but participation in society involves a compromise of freedom in order to promote the public good as well as the welfare of individual users.
- Radical approaches – where human beings are social beings whose freedom is realised in society, and where there needs to be individual and collective empowerment and a challenging of inequalities in the working for social change.

These writers perceive a development of **traditional values**:

- Respect for person – recognising each person as a unique individual. Acting: 'so act as to treat humanity, whether in your own person or that of any other, never solely as a means but always also as an end', (Kant quoted in Banks, 1995, p28).
- Protection – protecting the vulnerable when they are under threat from others or themselves.
- The purposeful expression of feelings – providing a safe environment for users or

carers to express their negative as well as positive feelings in a safe environment ;upholding those emotions so that, perhaps for the first time, the individual can consider and evaluate those emotions without the fear of condemnation or being overwhelmed by them.
- Acceptance – 'Acceptance is a principle of action wherein the caseworker perceives and deals with the client as he [sic] really is, including his strengths and weaknesses, with congenial and uncongenial qualities, his positive and negative feelings, his constructive and destructive attitudes and behaviour, maintaining all the while a sense of the client's innate dignity and personal worth',
                                           Biestek, 1976: p82.

A good example of this would be from the Macdonald and Sheldon Study (1997: p42) where one of the people interviewed comments: 'He (the social worker) doesn't always agree about my voices, and says 'no, it's your sickness'. I can talk to him about it. I feel quite comfortable discussing differences of opinion with him'.

Here, the social worker accepts the reality of the voices to the user, but also allows the individual to stand back from the voices and evaluate their reality and significance:

- Controlled emotional involvement – as the voluntary sector co-ordinator commented at the beginning of this chapter, social workers 'have a professionalism that offers a useful distance from the problem in hand and allows them to deal dispassionately with the situation'.
At the same time, as we've seen from the *Strategies for Living* research, users and carers need to feel that social workers are both genuine, and genuinely committed to working with them and in tune with their experience of their world.
- Non-judgemental attitude – clearly this does not mean shying away from making professional judgements. Also the worker needs to be clear with the people they are working with as to the consequences of their actions or proposed actions in relation to the effect on other people, society, the law etc.
- Client self-determination – as we've seen from the case example at the beginning of this chapter, an over-protective approach can in fact mean that individuals can become passive or conversely rebellious.

- Confidentiality – again, the issues around confidentiality will be subtly different for a worker in an agency setting, rather than working within a pure counselling model. This is especially so when issues of risk have to be addressed. The worker needs to be clear with the user as to what the limits of confidentiality are.
- Normalisation – a term which is often misunderstood and misused. It is based on assisting individuals to lead a valued, ordinary life. The founder of this approach, Wolfensberger, updated his approach and re-termed it 'social role valorisation' – seeking to enhance the perceived status of people with disabilities through their performance of socially desired and valued roles. (For a short summary, see Braye and Preston-Shoot, 1995: p39).
- Congruence – as we have seen before, it is most important, that the worker is seen as 'genuine'. The relationship between the worker and the user or carer is inevitably a power relationship. This power can be used to dominate or manipulate. Carl Rogers, the doyen of client-centred approaches, makes the powerful statement that:

It has been found that personal change is facilitated when the psychotherapist is what he [sic] is, when in the relationship with his client he is genuine and without 'front' or façade, openly being the feelings and attitudes which at the moment are flowing in him. We have coined the term 'congruence' to try to describe this condition.

Rogers, 1961: p61.

I once had the enlightening experience of buying a drink from a bar in an area where I had once practised as a social worker. The person serving had been a young person looked after by the local authority, and I had been one of her social workers. She gave me a succinct pen portrait of all her social workers, and the core of what she was saying was as to whether she had found the workers genuine, or as she described it, 'real' or not! Linda Hart's book (Hart, 1995) is an excellent example of power relationships in a mental health setting. For a fictional exploration of power, I would recommend Ursula LeGuin's *The Dispossessed* (Panther, 1976). Shevek, the hero, a philosopher scientist, finds himself in many ways in similar situations to a social worker, operating on the margins of complex individual social and political situations and with no instruments except the purposeful use of himself. LeGuin's final words in the book are:

'But he had not brought anything. His hands were empty, as they had always been', (p319).

Thompson, then, outlines a number of what he calls **'emancipatory values'**, (or **radical values**) which in a sense move the more traditional values forward in a world where it is increasingly recognised that individuals are part of a wider social and political milieu.

- De-individualisation – while recognising the uniqueness of the individual, there are merits in looking at connections and commonalities. Users can be seen in a wider context, particularly within the perspective of membership of oppressed groups. Thompson uses the example of working with a woman with depression, where the significance of gender can clearly be an issue with her concomitant expectations of female roles in current society (p117).
- Equality – a recognition and a willingness to confront inequalities.
- Social justice – although those social workers who advocated a greater voice for people in the institutions, and subsequently the closure and re-provision of the institutions, may not have recognised such actions as a pursuit of social justice, but that's what it was.
- Partnership – an increasing value put on this in government policies, in respect of engaging with users and carers and a range of agencies as equal partners in a shared enterprise.
- Citizenship – an idea we still seem to struggle with some thousands of years after the Greek city states developed the concept!

There were plenty of exceptions to citizenship in Greece, but we should have been able to move beyond that. Arguments for the extension of the franchise in Britain in the 19th and early 20th century now seem so self-evident. There is quite rightly an accent on rights and parallel responsibilities within the value of citizenship. But this should not be used as an excuse to deny care when that is required.

- Empowerment – this is both on an individual basis but also collectively. Both recognising the significance and recognising the severe disadvantages that pervade the everyday lives of people with mental health needs.
- Authenticity – recognising the boundary between those aspects of our lives that we can control and those that we cannot. In this, both

Figure 15: Values, relationships and constraints in the worker–user relationship.

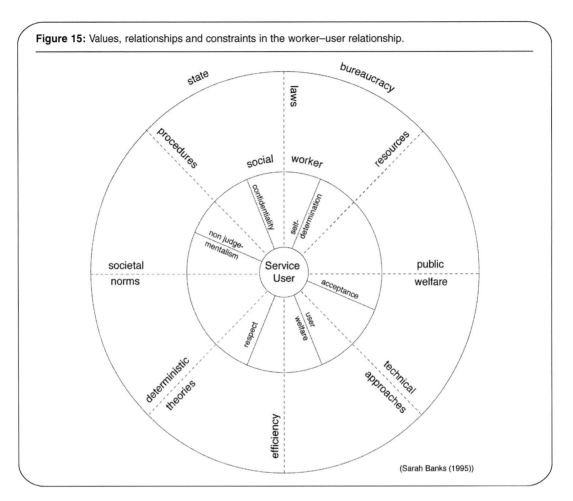

(Sarah Banks (1995))

the worker and the user or carers acknowledge the role they play and the responsibility they carry for their actions.

In 2002, the British Association of Social Workers reformulated the Statement of Principles and Principles of Practice which it had issued first in 1986. The booklet describes five basic values, and then outlines a number of principles attached to each value.
    These are:

- human dignity and worth
- social justice
- service to humanity
- integrity
- competence

There is then a section on ethical practice setting out guidance in particular situations:

- Responsibilities to service users:
  - priority of service user's interest
  - conflicts of interest
  - self-determination by service users
  - informed consent
  - services provided under compulsion
  - cultural awareness
  - privacy, confidentiality and records
- Responsibilities to the profession.
- Responsibilities in the workplace.
- Responses in particular roles:
  - management
  - education, training, supervision and evaluation
  - independent practice
  - research

A sound value-base is essential for a profession, for individual workers, for organisations and for the protection of vulnerable individuals who use services. Some, such as a commitment to recognising the humanity of each individual, must, I believe, be written in stone, others may ebb and flow in proportion to the type of agency and the state of society.

My voluntary sector contact, who is so positive about social work, also articulates the warning that when workers lose touch with their values and their own sense of self, then that hardness will be very hurtful to the user. Richard Titmus, the social philosopher, spoke movingly that:

> There cannot be one unambiguous goal for social work: human needs and desires are complex, interdependent, simultaneously rational and irrational and often in conflict. Nor is there one unambiguous objective for the social services. It would be terrifying if there were and if we thought there could be. All one is left with (or I am left with) is the philosopher's thought that increasing sensitiveness to the claims of others (and claims which cannot be wholly satisfied on the material criteria of the market) is one important element in the definition of moral progress in society.

Knowledge, skills and tasks

> Integrity without knowledge is weak and useless, and knowledge without integrity is dangerous and dreadful.
> Dr Johnson.

> What changes, are the social factors that cause these problems to persist or recur. Social work has to remain sensitive to these and to continually adapt its methods and techniques in order to deal with them. Victories may never by final but neither are the defeats.
> Sir William Utting, former Chief Social Work Officer, DHSS, *Professional Social Work*, 2002: p10.

> Social work as a profession has often been divided between a focus on individuals (casework) on the one hand, and on groups and communities (group work and community work) on the other. It also tended to suffer from a schism between social work educators and researchers, representing 'theory' on the one hand and the practitioners, representing 'practice' on the other hand.
> Professor Shulamit Ramon, Conference Paper, 27th April 2001.

> It is one thing to show a man he is in error and another to put him in possession of the truth.
> John Locke, *Essay Concerning Human Understanding*, 1689.

The National Institute for Mental Health in England was launched in 2001 with a remit to 'Reshape services and practice in line with the evidence base bringing together the research, development and dissemination functions of Mental Health Services' (Department of Health, June 2001).

At the time of writing, NIMHE's first national conference is planned to take place in Newcastle upon Tyne in June 2001. It is an appropriate

place, bearing in mind that a few miles down the road at Jarrow, the Venerable Bede penned the first History of England in the 8th century. One of the most famous passages from Bede is when a Northumbrian thane likens human existence to the sparrow that flies in from the dark into a warm and lighted hall and then out into the dark again. As he remarks, human beings welcome those who can enlighten us about the passage of life and its meaning.

Social work, as Butrym points out, is an 'applied discipline' 'in the sense that relevant knowledge acquired is for direct use in the pursuit of its objectives'. It has always had an inferiority complex where knowledge is concerned, partly because, as we can see in this text, the range of user needs, government imperatives and social work tasks is such that a broad spread of knowledge is required, and social workers' qualification training, set at two years, is clearly only long enough to skim the surface of the theoretical base. Doctors, for example, not only have longer qualifying training, but have a greater investment in post qualifying training as well.

Not all of the self-abnegation is justified, however. In an applied discipline, experience reflected upon in an appropriate way is valued enormously by users and colleagues. As Taylor and White comment in their searching text: *Practising Reflexivity in Health and Welfare: Making Knowledge* (Taylor and White, 2000) they point to 'professional practice in health and welfare' being 'characterised by a greater degree of anxiety about its goals and outcomes. As we have seen, social workers have to deal with uncertainties much more than certainties, and too often the dominant answer to this uncertainty has been a technical, procedural, and often bureaucratic one', (Taylor and White, 2000: p4).

Progress is based on exploration; often the major improvements in human welfare (the discovery of penicillin, for example) are founded in accident rather than design. Human beings crave certainty, and modern society believes that there is always a magic pill for every ailment. At the time of writing, NICE have just approved the prescription of a new range of drugs which trials have shown assist people with schizophrenia, with reduced risk of side effects. Unfortunately there was little in the guidance on social care.

In some senses, we feel happier with the pronouncements of 'science': from the Latin scientia – knowledge, and from Latin and French root words meaning to know, but also to separate, and divide into separate parts. This is connected but different again from 'knowing', from Greek, Latin and old English roots: to come to know, to recognise. Knowledge, as Thomas Kuhn (Kuhn, 1962) asserts, is a series of paradigms which are developed and then challenged and replaced. The Greek philosopher, Socrates, asserted that wisdom is: 'knowledge of what it is one does not know', echoed in modern times by Popper's assertion that 'our ignorance grows with our knowledge', (see Butrym, 1976: p63 and Karl Popper, *The Logic of Scientific Discovery*, 1934).

For man science is not enough on its own because human beings do not simply come as one-size fits all. In the context of international management, Geert Hofstede has demonstrated that if a business person with considerable expertise fails to shape their knowledge to the culture of the country they are operating in, they are doomed to failure (Hofstede, 1980).

It is very clear that the general practitioner and psychiatrist most appreciated by service users and carers is someone who combines both the scientist and the artist. As Magee has expressed it in his writings on Karl Popper: 'the scientist and the artist, far from being engaged in opposed or incompatible activities, are both trying to extend the range of understanding and of experience by the use of creative imagination, subjected to critical control. They both use irrational as well as rational faculties in the pursuit of this objective; they are both exploring the unknown and trying to articulate the search and its findings; both are seekers after truth who make indispensable use of intuition' (Magee, 1973: p72).

Thompson indicates the danger, which is too often evident, of social workers remarking: 'I prefer to stick to practice' (Thompson, 2000: p72-3) and the problems which follow from this dichotomy between theory and practice.

In 2001, the government set up the Social Care Institute for Excellence (SCIE) with its three main functions:

- To review current knowledge about social care.
- To develop best practice guides based on that knowledge.
- To ensure that those guides contribute to positive practice and policy change.

SCIE recognises that knowledge comes from diverse sources, including from research,

service reviews and from the experience of people who use and who provide social care services. As Mike Fisher, Director of Analysis and Reviews, emphasises: 'it's not "what works" but "what works for whom and under what circumstances" ', (quoted in *Community Care*, 25th April 2002, p35).

As Professor Olive Stevenson once wryly commented:

> to try and build a social work house on the shifting sands of social science theory is asking for trouble. Social work should probably concentrate on erecting strong, portable, flexible tents rather than houses.
>
> Stevenson, 1971: p226.

The National Institute for Mental Health in England will have its Mental Health Research Network but also development centres based on the geography of the government offices for the regions (vital for engaging with the wider citizenship and social inclusion agenda) who will work alongside practitioners, integrating theory and practice.

Incidentally, when I did my CQSW course at Sussex University in the mid 1970s, the seminar running right the way through the course was one integrating theory and practice so that the student placements always related back to theoretical concepts and vice versa.

As the poet T. S. Eliot saw it: 'perceptions do not, in a really appreciative mind, accumulate as a mass, but form themselves as a structure', (quoted in Kermode, 1975), and of course in a pilgrim profession, this may well be Stevenson's 'tents' rather than houses. Hugh England, in *Social Work as Art*, quotes Bowers in saying that:

> The subject matter of social casework is the individual human being as he [sic] exists in reality, that is, in a total situation ... casework does not deal with some particular segment of the individual, but with the individual as a **whole person**' (my emphasis).
>
> England, 1986: p105.

Knowledge is one thing, how we use it is another; and I know that the times when I felt I have 'got it wrong' is when I have inappropriately used knowledge from one setting and imposed it on another, e.g. having worked in a community, multi-disciplinary team, and feeling I knew the issues well, I made presumptions about the operation and issues of another community team in another place. We therefore need to use knowledge through:

- Selection – what we need at any one time.
- Integration – interlinking different forms of knowledge and theory with practice.

- Reflection – thinking through our actions and their consequences.
- Reflexion – interrogating our previously taken-for-granted assumptions (Taylor and White, 2000).

Case Example 7

This case example looks at the issues for the mental health of an elderly couple. The social worker requires considerable knowledge about human development, the psychology and physiology of ageing; the cultural issues for a couple coming from the Ukraine, and the issues around oppression and its effects impacting on people both in the present and in the future.

The social worker, Alison Kilbride, demonstrates an ability to listen, to empathise, to assess, to liaise with a range of other staff, and co-ordinate complex care packages, to assess risk and have the courage to stick with a risky situation including the experience of aggression from the user.

Reprinted with kind permission from Community Care, 17th-23rd May, 2001.

Knowledge and skills

Truth lies in the quality of the user's experience of the service.

Jane Campbell, Chair, SCIE.

There is still an insufficient commitment to applied social science in NHS Psychiatry. At the level of the frontline practitioner that is exactly what the social worker can provide ... but social science has yet to realise its full potential as a contributor to the study and management of illness and disability because it lags a long way behind the more dominant biochemical framework as far as the strength of its theoretical underpinnings are concerned.

With acknowledgements of the need to re-humanise our patients, and of the shortcomings of our current treatments, mental health services are faced with the challenge of embracing social science in a way that they haven't to date.

consultant psychiatrist.

The body of knowledge that social workers need to become proficient in consists of:

- Human development – the increasing accent on specialising and sub-specialties, means that sound knowledge on human development is more than ever important for

helping to understand the individual and the individual's family.
- Social processes and power dynamics – as we have seen in previous chapters, the construction of society, power dynamics within or outside institutions, and the issues of race and culture, bear heavily on the individual and their relationship with the world around them (see Thompson, 1998; Westwood et al., 1989; Fernando, 1995). In a case example, Suki Desai and Aasra Garib (1998) demonstrate how in inter-cultural situations in mental health the worker has a complex role of 'social interpreter' from the individual to the family, and vice versa, and from the individual and family to the other professionals involved so as to get round the cultural incomprehensibility that pertains.
- Social policy – not only what is but why and how it has developed.
- Law and constitution.
- Interpersonal and group dynamics.
- How organisations function.
- The value base – and how it works in practice.
- Theoretical paradigms:
  - psycho dynamics
  - psychosocial casework
  - humanistic psychology
  - behavioural
  - systems theory
  - radical approaches
  - participatory approaches
  - emancipatory practice

Methods of intervention

Methods of intervention are likely to follow closely on from theoretical perspectives and may include:

- Client-centred approaches – based on the work of Carl Rogers and Gerard Egan, starting where the person is, and moving from exploration to understanding, and then to action followed by evaluation.
- Task-centred practice where Reid and Shyne's work pointed to the benefits of short-term goals to boost self-esteem rather than an open ended therapeutic relationship.
- Crisis intervention – rather like judo (!), using the energy inherent in a crisis to move forward.
- Behavioural work – based on the work of behaviourists such as Skinner, and developed by social learning theorists, e.g. Albert Bandura, who 'emphasised that learning

Case Example 7

Rights and wrongs

An older couple with deteriorating physical and mental health and poor command of English provided social worker Alison Kilbride with the tough task of co-ordinating different agencies to ensure the couple's health and well being while respecting their human rights.

Case notes

Social worker: Alison Kilbride

Field: Senior practitioner in a mental health specialist team for older people Location: Oxfordshire social services

Client: Jak Navard (not his real name) is in his 80s and has progressive dementia. He lives with his wife, who has had a stroke, which resulted in physical and cognitive deterioration. Both were anti-fascist activists in eastern Europe during the war, and have English as a second language.

Case history: They were referred to the team when Mrs Navard was in hospital because of a stroke. A few days later her husband's mental confusion became evident to professionals. She was then sent to a rehabilitation unit for intensive physiotherapist and occupational therapist inputs. Mr Navard joined her because both became hostile when separated. She was discharged with a substantial community care package, and Kilbride's team arranged for a psychiatric assessment of Mr Navard, which confirmed progressive dementia. He began to exhibit paranoid behaviour towards care assistants and Kilbride, often refusing them access to his wife. They also stopped speaking and understanding English, as a result of which Ukranian interpreters were employed.

Then Kilbride and her colleagues were assaulted, which led to the care assistants being withdrawn. A subsequent psychiatric assessment confirmed the earlier diagnosis, changes were made in work practices to protect staff, and a mental health assertive outreach team employed to assist. They were admitted to a community hospital, and subsequently referred to a psychiatric assessment centre – the department of psychiatry and old age at a local mental health trust.

Dilemma: Their health and cognitive functioning is deteriorating, but they want to return home, and their wishes must be respected.

Risk factor: Even with an intensive care package, their health and safety is at risk.

Outcome: The centre wishes to discharge them back home.

The government's social care agenda with its emphasis on evidence-based practice and effective outcomes seems to have been broadly welcomed, despite continuing concerns about the future role of social services. But of course social workers are often faced with the difficult job of trying to sort what an effective outcome is. In many situations this is far from clear.

Alison Kilbride, a senior mental health practitioner in a specialist team for older people, is still grappling with this question in her work with Mr and Mrs Navard (not their real name). The couple, who are now in their 80s, suffered political persecution in the Ukraine prior to and during the Second World War, and came here as refugees many years ago. They were not known to statutory services until Mrs Navard had a stroke and was treated in hospital. At that time it became clear that she was malnourished and showed other signs of self-neglect, and two days later when their GP visited the husband, he admitted that he was becoming confused.

They were referred to the hospital social work department, and subsequently agreed to enter a rehabilitation unit, where she received intensive physiotherapy and where an occupational therapy assessment was made. It was noticed that the couple became hostile when separated.

The hospital social work department decided to refer the couple to Kilbride.

She says that it was clear to everyone that Mr Navard had progressive dementia, and that as a result of this and his wife's condition, they were at significant risk. Consequently, a substantial care package was put in place, and Kilbride and her colleagues arranged a psychiatric assessment for the Navards. The assessment confirmed that they were suffering from progressive dementia. Meanwhile, their home had been thoroughly cleaned, and adaptations made to assist Mrs Navard, who had significant physical impairments.

The couple had expressed a wish to remain in their own home, and at first the care package, which included many personal care services for Mrs Navard, appeared to be working. But then her husband started to exhibit paranoid symptoms. He began to make it difficult for the care assistants to attend to his wife, and at times refused entry to them, to Kilbride and to the community psychiatric nurse, all of whom had been visiting very regularly. Also, at about this time he began to be unable to understand or speak English, and she subsequently arranged for Ukrainian interpreters to visit alongside the care staff in an effort to persuade him to allow them to attend to her. Kilbride had offered the couple the option of residential care, but this had been rejected. Malnourishment was now becoming a major concern.

Meanwhile, the state of their home was deteriorating to such an extent that rats were often seen, and on more than one occasion the Navards' deteriorating cognitive functioning caused safety problems, for example the microwave oven had burst into flames.

Consequently, a case conference was called, and a decision was made to intensify the care package, basically to ensure that one carer could distract Mr Navard while the other attended to his wife. Additional attention was given to ways in which the daily visitors, namely Kilbride, the community practice nurse and the care assistants, could act to ameliorate his 'very excitable' state. She had also engaged an assertive outreach team from the local NHS department of old age and psychiatry to help.

Shortly after this, and despite these efforts, Kilbride and her colleagues were assaulted by one or other of the couple, as a result of which the care agency withdrew their staff. 'This happened to me despite the presence of a Ukrainian-speaking interpreter, because by now Mr Navard was unable to recognise me. Thankfully, my manager and others in the authority supported me a great deal after the assault, but we had obviously reached another crisis,' she says. Consequently, the couple did not have the support of care assistants for a few weeks. In the meantime, Kilbride had contacted the GP, who the couple still trusted, in the hope that he would arrange another psychiatric assessment, she also asked the same of the assertive outreach service.

'By this time the various agencies had already decided that compulsory admission under the Mental Health Act 1983 was inappropriate, even though it was clear that their health was deteriorating and the risks to their safety were increasing,' she says.

The GP persuaded the Navards to enter a community hospital so that their physical health could be attended to, but while they were there their behaviour deteriorated rapidly and a decision was made to transfer them to a psychiatric assessment centre. The centre has now decided that they should be discharged back to their home.

'I'm now faced with them returning home, with only a minimal amount of care assistance, which I've managed to secure from another care agency. There are enormous health and safety risks, which are also recognised by the community practice nurse and the psychiatrist, but there are no legal means to avoid this situation. I am investigating the use of an electronic keypad on their front door, so that access can be assured, although I'm concerned about the human rights implications of taking this step. I'm keeping all the agencies informed about what's happening, and exploring residential and nursing home options,' she says.

'I'm terribly concerned about both of them, and particularly about Mrs Navard's health and her very low quality of life,' Kilbride concludes.

Arguments for risk

- Mr and Mrs Navard have always stated that they wish to remain together in their own home.
- Suitable residential or nursing home care facilities are hard to identify, given the couple's loss of English, and his paranoid behaviour.
- A co-ordinated approach by care staff, members of the assertive outreach service, and their GP, could help to secure and operate a new care package.
- It may be possible under Mental Health Act 1983 provisions to put Mr Navard on a medication regime, which would ameliorate his paranoid behaviour, although the department of psychiatry and old age would need to be in full agreement.
- Social services, with the Navards' agreement, administers their finances.

Arguments against risk

- Mrs Navard's health is at serious risk unless she receives regular assistance in washing, feeding and other personal care.

- Both of them are living in squalid conditions, and their behaviour creates serious risks to their personal safety.
- The state of their home is beginning to impact on neighbours, and there is a likelihood that the environmental health service will be called in, which would undoubtedly create further distress.
- Their increasingly aggressive behaviour could lead to care staff being injured.
- They are socially isolated, and now unable to use English, which effectively precludes the option of organising any wider support, befriending or other care network to underpin statutory services.
- Their progressive dementia, allied to their personal histories, make it ever more likely that they will view the intrusion into their lives of care services as a threat.

Independent comment

The challenges here are enormous. Kilbride has done an admirable job in trying to maintain an isolated older couple in the community who have both physical and mental difficulties and specific cultural needs, *write Alisoun Milne and Jayne Lingard.* The key risks are around the safety of Mr and Mrs Navard and also the safety of the care staff. Despite the best efforts of Kilbride, the couple remain very vulnerable and have retreated into a world that isolates them from help and support.

Although use of the Mental Health Act 1983 has been considered, a formal risk assessment that takes account of Mr Navard's dementia has not been conducted. This may help decision making by locating risk in a coherent framework that respects user rights and applies the principles of person-centred care. A jointly administered risk assessment, which takes account of the needs of both Mr and Mrs Navard, may be helpful.

Although an interpreter has been employed, we do not know if this person has any understanding of the nature of dementia. An advocate trained in communicating with people with dementia may help the Navards to make informed decisions about their future care.

The Navards and Kilbride have been failed by the separate delivery of health and social care services, and the even wider gap between the care of people's physical health and their mental health. The couple were assessed in a number of settings and by a range of social and health care teams. Neither the Audit Commission's report on mental health services for older people with mental health needs[1] nor standard seven of the National Service Framework for Older People[2] directly confront the current pattern of services failing to meet the needs of the whole person.

Alisoun Milne and **Jayne Lingard** are consultants to the Mental Health Foundation's programme of work on Mental Health in Later Life and are both qualified social workers.

[1] Audit Commission, *Forget-Me-Not: Mental Health Services for Older People*, Audit Commission, 2000
[2] DoH, National Service Framework for Older People, March 2001

Reprinted by kind permission of *Community Care*, 17–23 May, 2001.

behaviour is a social act, acquired through modelling, imitation and observation' (Pierson in Hanvey and Philpot, 1994, p83).

- Radical emancipatory intervention – based on confronting oppressive social structures.
- Care management – the procurement, delivery, monitoring and evaluation of care packages (see below).
- Advocacy – but professional workers need to be very aware that there are a number of times when it is inappropriate for the professional to act as advocate, and an independent advocate needs to be brought in. As a service user once remarked to me: 'I have an excellent social worker, she battles on my behalf, but she and I are both aware that she works for social services, and sometimes I need somebody who works just for me.'

For greater detail and more exploration of the issues see Thompson, 2000; Coulshead and Orme, 1998; Hanvey and Philpot, 1994.

Skills and tasks

The former Central Council for the Education and Training of Social Workers (CCETSW) published a set of competencies for social work students in respect of the Diploma in Social Work (which replaced the Certification of Qualification in Social Work and the Certificate in Social Services). The 1996 version sets out the competencies under six headings:

1. Communicate and engage – with users and carers, colleagues and partner organisations.
2. Promote and enable – 'promote opportunities for people to use their own strengths and expertise to enable them to meet their responsibilities, secure rights and achieve change', (CCETSW, 1996: p11).
3. Assess and plan.
4. Intervene and provide services.
5. Work in organisations.
6. Develop professional competence.

Social workers have retreated from the social model, as they experience difficulties in finding a voice.
consultant psychiatrist with a strong emphasis on social perspectives.

Anti-oppressive practice is not an area which has a great deal of impact in Health Service thinking. It is imperative that social workers continue to strive to achieve this and challenge when it is not happening.
social worker in a multi-disciplinary team.

Skills are intrinsically linked with the values, the humanity and human construct of the individual, and the knowledge base.

It clearly helps if the worker has innate human skills of being integrated (in terms both of personal integrity and self-belief), sensitivity, open-mindedness, patience and being well organised. In fact, recent research by the Sainsbury Centre (Murray et al., 1997 and Maca, 2002) demonstrate that the innate qualities of the support workers, their trust-worthiness, caring attitudes and availability were more important to users than professional qualifications. e.g.

I can talk to her, she's normal – there's no professional fence, no prying and less making me do things. I do things for her because of the way she approaches it. If things are hard for me to do, then I know she will be there to help. It's not just, 'do this because I say so and maybe I'll help', which you get from professionals. They give less pressure and far less criticism.
Murray et al., 1997: p44.

The skills I describe below, however, are not theoretical, but ones I have seen demonstrated by social workers I have worked for, worked with and managed. Social work education, if it's effective, should be able to build on, consolidate, enhance and sharpen existing skills, and develop new skills, (Thompson, 2000, Chapter 4):

Self-awareness

Awareness of the user's history, hopes, fears, abilities, needs, aspirations etc.

Awareness of our own formative influences, preconceptions etc.

How we come across to users and carers.

How external factors affect us, e.g. I once managed a heroic and very skilled unqualified social worker, who had been placed, in my view quite irresponsibly, within an organisational minefield of an institution, with no adequate support. Her supervisor, social work trained, had never overcome his fear of and distaste for institutions, and therefore rarely set foot in the hospital to support her and to battle for the rights of the individuals within the institution.

Self-management

'Good people skills', writes Neil Thompson, 'have their root in personal effectiveness' (Thompson, 1996: p7).

The ideal helper for Gerard Egan 'realises that he [sic] must model the behaviour he hopes to help others achieve. He knows that he can help only if, in the root sense of the term, he is a 'potent' human being, a person with the will and the resources to act' (Egan, 1975: p22).

The workers must be able to manage themselves, their time and their record keeping.

Resilience is also important and workers must strive to ensure that they do not become over-stressed and that they preserve a work-life balance, (see Gilbert and Thompson, 2002: p97–107).

> *With the realisation of one's own potential and self-confidence in one's ability, one can build a better world.*
> The Dalai Lama.

Communication skills

One of the earliest management texts in the post Roman western world has the line: 'listen with the ear of the heart' (Benedict of Nursia, 540 AD) and the skill of listening, hearing, responding and then acting is a fundamental social work facility. Too passive a listening or jumping in too quickly with proposed actions undermines the user or carer.

Communication skills need to be both verbal and non-verbal (attempting to listen while seated behind a desk with your arms folded does not normally denote receptivity!). Written skills in reports for courts, tribunals, communication with other agencies etc. is a vital function when representing a user, as is also technical facility with phones, emails etc.

Analytical skills

Identifying key issues, and sifting the important items from the accumulation of facts which often cloud rather than clarify the issue.

Identifying patterns and acting to check these out and connect them.

As Noel and Rita Timms urged in an early social work text ' . . . acceptance should describe the active search to discover *the point*', (Timms and Timms, 1997: p88).

Analytical skills, then, need to be brought forward in all elements of the helping process from working with the user to explore their world, helping to create patterns which assist, planning actions and reviewing them.

Sensitivity and observational skills

Empathy with the individual.

Identifying issues of culture, gender, race, position and role, and other power-related factors and acting to address these.

Reflection

A constant reflection on practice and challenge to our existing presumptions and practices (see Taylor and White, 2000).

Handling feelings

Acquaintances sometimes say 'Well social work is just about listening to people, isn't it? We all do that', but when they see the strength, sometimes the violence of the emotional inter-play, they usually change their mind. As Donald Winnicott pointed out in his influential 1963 work, *Casework and Mental Illness*, part of the social work role is one of 'holding', staying with the individual through many trials and tribulations. It is this 'stickability' which Macdonald and Sheldon point to as one of the most helpful factors in the Westminster Study.

Planning and co-ordination

This aspect of work has been sharpened by care management (although not all social workers would agree with this!) and one can see a change in emphasis in Gerard Egan's work as he moves from his 1975 version of *The Skilled Helper*, to the 7th edition in 2002. Timms and Timms pointed out that in the 1970s, workers sometimes seem to have been 'so preoccupied with understanding a situation that they have not been free enough to do much to change it', (Timms and Timms, 1977: p100) but Winnicott in 1963 was quite clear that 'integration is vitally important in this connection, and your (social workers) work is quite largely counteracting disintegrating forces in individuals and in families and in localised social groups' (Winnicott, 1963: p227).

Partnership skills

'What service users value', writes Professor Peter Beresford, Professor of Social Policy, and Director of the UK Centre for Citizen Partnership at Brunel University, and a long-term user, 'are participatory ways of working, whether in the production of services, support or knowledge. It is not a question of reducing the role of other stakeholders, but of ensuring service users are routinely included among them and have opportunities to speak for themselves and offer their own discussions on equal terms. Service users must be involved and included in *everything* from the start and at every stage' (Beresford, 2002: p16).

George Bernard Shaw once remarked that 'all professions are a conspiracy against the laity' and this can be as true of social work as any other profession. The voluntary sector service co-ordinator who was so positive about social work in an earlier part of the text also remarked:

'There is a real need to meet each client with an open mind and listen hard to what they are saying – the solution is probably very deep within their words'. 'There is a tendency to go with the history of the client when they might have changed, or the history might have been written by someone who wasn't listening properly' (voluntary sector, service co-ordinator in conversation with the author, May 2002).

Creativity

Some people are naturally creative, but creativity in the helping professions will develop from active listening to individuals and reflection on practice, either individually or in groups.

One of the main benefits of multi-disciplinary working should be increased creativity – if it isn't, we should be asking why not!

Presentation skills

Social work inevitably means assisting a user in presenting their case for resources, benefits, or in a legal/para-legal situation, or presenting on their behalf.

Presentational skills are not only important in formal situations but discussions with influential others. The approved social worker not only has to have knowledge and skills but has to argue their case influentially with those who have more overt organisational power than they do.

In conclusion, as we can see, these are skills which are in some sense technical, but by no means *just* technical. If they are simply a mechanical working out of techniques, then the individual being worked with will readily spot that. As Bill Jordan puts it:

*In suggesting that to be helpful the helper must be a real person, I am making it clear that I think helping is not simply a skill or expertise or technique. Helping is a test for helper as a person. It involves the disciplined use of the **whole** of the personality . . . he has also to retain his own values and standards, his own strengths and virtues. He has to recognise that the other person's feelings and fantasies are real to him, and to share in the discomfort of them, yet also to stay in touch with his own reality.*
Jordan, 1979: p26 (my emphasis).

Or as Winnicott colourfully puts it:

They (the users) take a risk, and first they must test you to see if you may be able to prove sensitive and reliable or whether you have it in you to repeat the traumatic experiences of their past. In a sense, you are a frying pan, with the frying process played backwards, so that you really do unscramble the scrambled eggs.
Winnicott, 1963: p227.

Perhaps the main fault is that social workers feel they have to resolve things. They are needed by the client to listen, respond effectively and sensitively and then to come up with some practical measures to alleviate some aspects of the problem. The punter knows that social workers are not miracle workers, but they need a professional person to help them through the mire and to access useful support in order to move forward.
voluntary sector service co-ordinator.

Social work support

The key contributions made by the social worker to the support package are: care planning skills to co-ordinate a multi-agency and cross service package. The stability to provide ongoing professional support over a number of years, enabling good relationships to be built and engagement with long-term aims. A person-centred focus to ensure that the client's needs are met when they do not fit established service provision. Local knowledge is used to provide practical support, e.g. pay as you go leisure facilities. Professional support has overcome stressful crises, e.g. burglaries and flat moves.

The tasks for social workers are:

Assessment

This is an assessment looking at the whole person in the context of their close relationships, family, community, neighbourhood, culture and faith, past experiences, future aspirations, strengths and needs (see Figures 5 and 10 above).

As the 1959 Younghusband report stated:

We regard the essential functions of social workers in the Health and Welfare Services as being to assess the disturbance of equilibrium in a given' individual 'and his (sic) family and social relationships so as to give appropriate help. The aim will be to offer a supporting relationship in which his and their fears, frustrations and anxieties are understood, and measures used to meet or lessen them.

Younghusband, 1959.

The user is essentially the 'owner' of their own 'story'. Butler and Pritchard are clear

Case Example 8

Brief history

John H is in his mid-thirties and has experienced schizophrenic illness since his teenage years. Six years ago he was admitted to hospital under Section following an episode of self-mutilation. He expressed a strong wish to live in his own flat on discharge and has spent the last six years living independently with a support package co-ordinated through the care programme approach, with a multi-disciplinary team providing ongoing professional support.

Current situation

John rents his own council flat with daily visits from a home care agency to provide practical support around budgeting, meal preparation, medication and maintaining the flat. Members of the multi-disciplinary team meet with John every six weeks to review the support package and work with any arising difficulties. For example, harassment from a neighbour or falling out with a support worker. The high level of support has been felt appropriate because John's levels of motivation, concentration and self-worth mean that self-neglect is a significant risk.

John is offered some structured day activities. In the past, he used a day centre but with growing independence, it became increasingly clear that this provision was inappropriate and John could receive a better day service from mainstream services. John now attends one group session with a day service for people with disabilities because he particularly likes the session, has someone to work with him on a one-to-one basis for recreational community activities and is beginning to engage with sessional groups with a mental health day service.

John is someone with a dual diagnosis of mental health needs and a mild learning disability. There is always the risk that he may fall between services and not receive proper support around his mental distress from either learning disability or mental health services. The support package that John has recognises this dilemma by providing day care which he feels is appropriate, while ensuring that he has ongoing support to develop his daily living skills.

that the 'social worker should be conscious of the potential strengths that exist within client and family, as well as apparent weaknesses and areas of dysfunction (Butler and Pritchard, 1983:, p43); and the report into the care and treatment of Christopher Clunis, remarked on the fact that the strengths that the family had had to offer were never properly brought into play, (Ritchie et al., 1994).

Smale, Tuson and Statham describe a number of types of assessment process, and look closely at what they call the 'questioning model' and the 'exchange model'.

The Questioning Model

Assumes the worker:

- Is expert in people and their needs.
- Exercises knowledge and skill to form their own assessment to identify people's needs.
- Identifies resources required.
- Takes responsibility for making an accurate assessment of need and taking appropriate action.

The Exchange Model

Assumes that people are expert in themselves.

Assumes that the worker:
- Has expertise in the process of problem-solving with others.
- Understands and shares perceptions of problems and their management.
- Gets agreement about who will do what to support whom.
- Takes responsibility for arriving at the optimum resolution of problems within the constraints of available resources and the willingness of participants to contribute.

Smale et al., 2000: p140.

Working towards positive change

As we have seen already, social work operates at the margins of society, and is often in the position of interpreting the user's world to members of his/her family, groups and professionals, and conversely, interpreting the outside world and various groups and cultures to the user.

Egan's latest development of the skilled helper model has three stages:

1. What's going on? Telling the story, looking at 'blind spots' and considering leverage.

Figure 16: Assessing the individual's needs in their historical context.

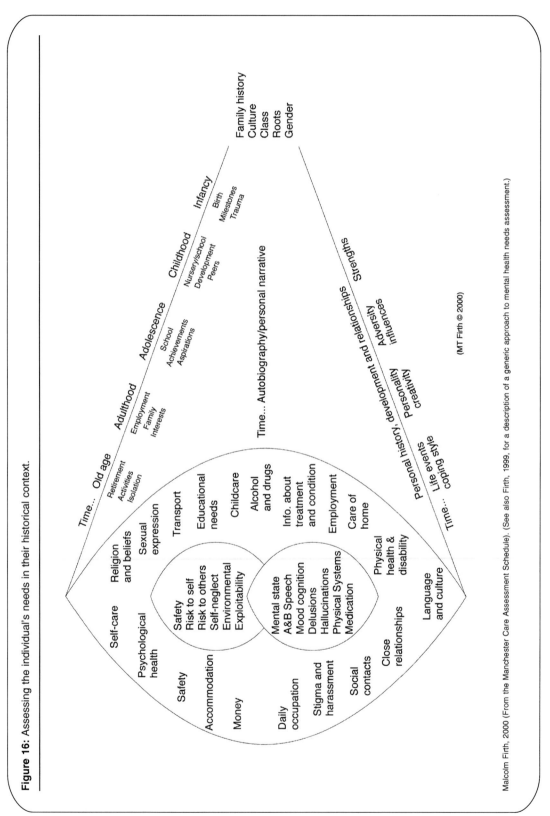

(MT Firth © 2000)

Malcolm Firth, 2000 (From the Manchester Care Assessment Schedule). (See also Firth, 1999, for a description of a generic approach to mental health needs assessment.)

2. What solutions make sense for the user? Possibilities – change agendas and commitment to change.
3. How does the user get what they need or want? Possible strategies – best fit plan.

The social worker will arrive on the scene at a time of crisis, as can be seen by most of the case examples in this text, and therefore 'no change' is very rarely an option, while change without consent, participation, empowerment and self-direction will cause problems with self-determination later on.

> *Every day social workers help people from all walks of life, connecting thousands of people to appropriate resources. Social workers help people understand their own personal power to overcome life's adversities.*
> Elizabeth Clarke, Executive Director, National Association of Social Workers, USA quoted in Snell, *What About the Social Workers?* ADSS Inform, 11: 1, April 2002.

Ongoing support

Martin Davies sees one of social work's prime tasks as: 'contributing to the maintenance and growth of those citizens seen to be deprived and underprivileged, and trying to enrich the lives of those on the margins of society.' (Davies, 1981).

It is one of the features of social work that many workers' fears have been neglected following the introduction of care management in 1993, which had a greater emphasis on short-term interventions and co-ordinating practical care packages with a lesser emotional component.

The Westminster Study is essential reading to understand how vital the ongoing support is for people with multiple social and environmental needs and environmental as well as personal needs, and as one colleague in the voluntary sector said to me recently 'Who else is going to deal with the nitty gritty of life?'

Planning, monitoring and review

This can be a cycle of interventions, on a partnership basis, around behaviours and interactions, and/or the bringing into play of packages of care (see also Care Management below) which is a feature of a number of the case examples in this text where users are particularly vulnerable and there are major elements of risk.

Co-ordinating

The world doesn't get any simpler! One of the prime tasks of the social worker is to co-ordinate work across a number of professional disciplines and agencies so as to ensure that the user is in as much control of the situation as is possible, they are not subject to multi individual consultations or subject to the oppressive posse of professionals; while at the same time ensuring that all the professionals and agencies deliver.

Information gathering

One of the universal rules of information is that one is always overwhelmed with a plethora when one doesn't need it, but accurate and understandable information is not around when you do.

Because of their social perspective and links with a wide range of social agencies, social workers are in a good position to gather information or signpost.

When I was researching the needs of carers with disabled offspring in West Sussex in the early 1980s, one of the major pleas was for better information. We produced an information handbook, which one parent described as 'A real hand of friendship' (conversation with the author).

Nowadays, information changes so rapidly that a careful judgement has to be made as to whether information is printed or produced for electronic distribution. Issues of race, culture and language are, of course, crucial as has already been mentioned earlier in the text (see Fernando, 1995).

Empowerment

The social work task is to empower the people we work with, and to ensure that issues of citizenship, rights and empowerment are at the forefront of other professionals working with users and carers.

Linda Hart's autobiographical work, *Phone at Nine Just to Say You're Alive* (Hart, 1997) is a powerful description of the issues around power relationships between users and professionals. See also works such as Harding and Beresford, 1996.

Education

All professions should be a source of education for colleagues and other agencies in the values,

Table 4: The social work contribution to mental health services.

Knowledge	Skills	Ethics
Mental health, Social welfare, family and human rights law. Sociology. Social administration. Social and individual psychology. Social philosophy and the ethics of social welfare. Social work methods. Models of social intervention and empowerment. Research. Race, gender, and disability studies.	Individual and family casework. Group work. Social brokerage, mediation, and advocacy skills. Advocacy. Use of relationship as an enabling process. The assessment of a person's social circumstances and needs, and communication of the conclusions. The compilation of assessment reports for specific purposes. Assessments regarding the potential need for compulsory detention and treatment under the Mental Health Act. The co-ordination and implementation of community care packages. The evaluation of complex needs on a more general level to assist planning and development. Advising fellow professionals on the relevance of social factors. Reflective analysis.	All that is included in the BASW Code of Ethics including the following commitments: • To a distinct set of professional principles and values based on the worth and the social and civil rights of each individual and groups as an integral part of the work. • To anti-discriminatory and anti-oppressive practice. • Commitment to promoting and upholding self determination and social inclusion. • To the least restrictive alternative. • Commitment to ongoing learning and professional development.

Table compiled by the Mental Health Special Interest Group, a National Forum representing Social Work in Mental Health. From the BASW Website, May 2002.

strengths, knowledge and skills which they have.

While social workers sometimes have a lack of confidence in this, the emphasis on a social and community agenda in the United Kingdom at present should give them confidence in espousing and propounding the social perspective.

In all of this, it should never be forgotten that the social worker is working alongside the most vulnerable people in our society at the margins of identity, recognition and tolerance, and in situations of conflict, distress and paradox.

There is often an underlying assumption in public life that another structural change, procedure or initiative will reduce 'the complexity, ambiguity and uncertainty inherent in the workers' pivotal position'.

A more realistic position is to recognise this lack of certainty as an inevitable and integral dimension of the role of the social change agent. The task is to balance these different perceptions and reconcile conflicting behaviours. Ambiguity, confusion and complexity are not problems to be solved before the job can be done: working towards their resolution is the work.

Smale et al., 2000: p94.

If I were to summarise my reflections, it would be to encourage you to be bold, and emphasise not only the statutory and supportive contributions social work can make to Mental Health Services, but to come out of the shadows, so to speak, and emphasise the intellectual contribution as well.

consultant psychiatrist.

Social work and care management

Social work is providing relationships to people in the context of their systems, to help them best negotiate complex decisions and transitions.

Professor Andrew Cooper.

There isn't time here to go into the whys and wherefores of the NHS and Community Care Act, 1990, (implemented 1st April 1993). The tensions between the increasing numbers of vulnerable people requiring care and an escalating social security bill; between the Treasury and 10 Downing Street; the ambitions and fears of both the NHS and local authorities; and the challenge to simultaneously promote choice while keeping a lid on the pot of available resources, is a complex seesaw well set out in Lewis and Glennerster's *Implementing the New Community Care*, (1996).

Lewis and Glennerster's conclusion is that:

They (the reforms) were not primarily driven by a desire to improve the relations between the various statutory authorities, or to improve services for elderly people, or to help those emerging from mental hospital. They were driven by the need to stop the haemorrhage in the social security budget and to do so in a way that would minimise political outcry and not give additional resources to the local authorities themselves.
                                                                p8.

The new care managers, or those social workers re-designated care managers, were the people who had the creative role of assessing individual needs and creating care packages out of the former social security money transferred to social services under the Special Transitional Grant, and simultaneously balancing those individual needs with the amount of money available.

'Choice' was a word on everybody's lips, yet as Lewis and Glennerster point out:

The new policy was precisely designed to ration that choice in order to save public money. The right to be assessed and sensitive care management that would take account of everyone's preferences, including carers, seemed a way of squaring the circle. The difficulty was that circles have the rather irritating property of not being squares!
                    Lewis and Glennerster, 1996: p14.

There is no doubt that care managers did in fact make far better use of the social security money, in retaining people's independence, and re-abling those who had been admitted to institutions of various kinds. At the same time, finances were never adequate, some authorities running out within the first year, and therefore, to quote one Director of Social Services: 'social workers have become the public face of denial'.

Lewis and Glennerster's studies of a number of different kinds of authorities found some people feeling that 'it would erode much valued aspects of social work practice.' (p141) 'turn them into administrators and financial processors' (p140). But there were also numerous occasions when social workers/care managers found that they could produce positive outcomes for the users and carers they were working with, through the budgets delegated to them or their team managers, rather than scraping together resources from a whole range of different agencies.

The process of care management, as set down by the Department of Health Care Management and Assessment Guides in 1991 show a great deal of congruence with the social work task described above.

Social workers feared, however, that the therapeutic aspects of their role would be eroded, and in fact some social services departments did appear to see the advent of community care as a way of moving away from that particular aspect of the work; while others integrated the process with traditional social work; and others again split social work and care management. The parallel issue of whether nurses wished to take on the care management role in addition to their therapeutic one is mirrored today in the debate over the 'Approved Mental Health Practioner' role as proposed in the reform of the 1983 Mental Health Act (see Chapter 6).

In many cases, there seems to have been a misunderstanding as to what people like Challis at the PSSRU envisaged care management to be. Challis and his colleagues in fact made a distinction between 'administrative' and 'complete' care management (or case management). They wrote:

It is possible to define a rather limited form of case management -described here as 'administrative' case management – where service arrangements and co-ordination are seen as the central tasks. The other tasks of case management such as counselling, dealing with psychological stresses and tensions arising from caring or providing advice to families would be undertaken by persons other than the case manager . . . An underlying weakness in the 'administrative' model of case manage-ment is the failure to recognise the nature of the responsibilities and decisions which have to be made by the case manager.
                        Challis et al., 1990: p15
                        (see also Smale et al., 1994).

My belief is that it simply isn't sensible to separate care management and social work. My own experience as a social worker and as a manager, added to the research, leads me to the conclusion that users and carers need and want attention to *both* their emotional/psychological needs and their practical concerns, in a way which values them as unique individuals. Social work and care management are two sides of the same coin. Social workers who veer too much towards a counselling perspective, and do not address the practical needs of users or combat oppression, are in danger of pathologising the individual. Those who only address practical concerns are in danger of dehumanising the individual so that the whole process becomes caricatured as a package, whereby the user is

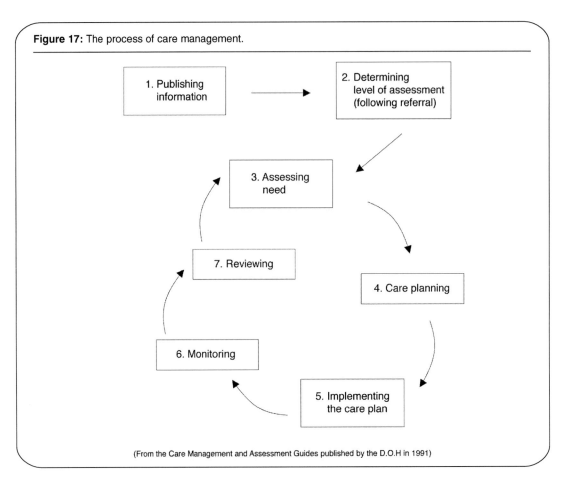

Figure 17: The process of care management.

1. Publishing information

2. Determining level of assessment (following referral)

3. Assessing need

7. Reviewing

4. Care planning

6. Monitoring

5. Implementing the care plan

(From the Care Management and Assessment Guides published by the D.O.H in 1991)

processed and 'boxed' in a way that denies them their dignity and uniqueness.

The Staffordshire approach, set down in the policy and practice guidelines, integrated social work and care management with a focus on users and carers, but the department was also very clear with those it served, and those it worked with as partners, that resources were finite.

The Westminster Study, conducted three years after the implementation of Community Care demonstrates again what some American commentators had already warned their English counterparts, namely that a purchaser/provider split within the main professionals delivering care (i.e. social workers/care managers) 'is an artificial macro construct which has nothing to do with micro practice in the human services and which is being imposed on a natural helping process', (Phyllis Sturgess, San Jose State University, in Clark and Lapsley, 1996).

Macdonald and Sheldon demonstrate clearly that:

Clients value the opportunity to discuss and clarify their worries and fears, and examine ways of overcoming them ('emotional support and reassurance'). This important aspect of service provision has been shown to be one that needs protecting within current organisation changes towards a purchaser/provider split and privatisation. The growing pressure here is to purchase what is easy to define and to monitor what it is easy to count, whether or not those inputs have a close 'logical fit' with the qualitative nature of clients' problems.
                    Macdonald and Sheldon, 1997: p43.

The Sainsbury Centre Study on Care Management in Mental Health quoted a range of reactions, but several positive ones are worth quoting:

I think the advantage of care management is that it brings a structure to the social work process.

I wish assessment and care management had come in twenty-five years ago, because it would have made me a better social worker.

'... the creative professional can mould together different traditions and approaches so as to improve their practice.

As one experienced senior manager put it in Staffordshire 'We're still doing social work but we are doing it in a more organised, systematic and effective way'.

Some of the same difficulties in melding together two strands of work, reappeared in the requirements and difficulties in merging care management and the care programme approach.

I will leave the last word to Macdonald and Sheldon:

> The role of specialist social workers was obviously pivotal in the system of care. They both arranged for services, and were a service themselves (an awkward principle for those who speak and write about 'services', as if these were always 'things'). In this study, the social services staff emerged as individuals to be relied upon, to promote emotional support and counselling, for a range of practical services, and for their well-respected 'advocacy' function. This appears to have been carried out with a distinctive friendliness, openness and professionalism which, for the majority of respondents, was thought to be the best thing about the help they received.
>
> p51.

The social worker in the community mental health team

> Mental health issues have predominantly been within the domain of psychiatry, concentrating on mental ill-health rather than mental health. This approach is in the process of being cemented further in the 'ill-health' camp with the movement of social work to the NHS. The NHS has traditionally spent many millions on reacting to ill-health and relatively little on maintaining health and social well-being. I am of the opinion that psychiatry should be an adjunct to social inclusion and social support for those suffering from mental health problems, rather than the lead profession. The role, training and model of social care within psychiatry needs to be enhanced greatly if the traditional view of mental ill-health being a lifetime problem is going to be challenged. Social workers are in a great position to influence this challenge but the overall philosophy needs to be addressed by the policy makers and traditional psychiatric services.
>
> Director of Integrated Mental Health Services, from a nursing background.

I am profoundly disappointed when I come across community mental health teams where there seems to be more of a focus on inter-disciplinary rivalry than inter-disciplinary working. Clearly, forming a team (though sometimes the teams seem more like groups) – as Malcolm Payne's work demonstrates, is a complex process and the effective team needs to operate more like a creative football team, rather than like an athletics team concentrating on their own individual pursuits (see Payne, 1982).

When teams are not functioning properly, the following problems are mentioned frequently by staff:

- *Poor leadership, either providing no structure or control, or imposing an authoritarian style.*
- *Lack of clarity about roles and responsibilities within the team.*
- *Absence of or infrequent meetings.*
- *Poor communication about team functions, and between members of the team.*
- *Time not managed to enable members to meet.*
- *Opinions not sought and talents not recognised and used.*
- *Lack of training.*
- *Poor working conditions.*

Gilbert and Scragg, 1992: p158.

My disappointment stems partly from being part of a very positive community team for people with learning disabilities in the mid 1980s (see Gilbert and Spooner, 1982). The senior community nurse had been appointed to lead a community nursing team only, but he was quite clear that a multi-disciplinary approach would be better for the people we served, both users and carers, and would have a long-term positive effect for the working together of the two major statutory agencies; also creating better links with the voluntary sector.

Some of the features of the team were as follows:

- A very clear focus, at the outset, on producing positive outcomes for users and carers.
- A shared operational policy for the team with an explicit value-base.
- Right from the beginning, recognising and celebrating the strength and skills that each profession had to bring to the team.
- A lack of defensiveness about professional roles, but within the operational policy, being clear with ourselves and our clientele what the core roles of each profession were, and also what the positive overlaps were.
- An open referral system with an initial team discussion of each case referred, and an agreement over which worker/workers would work with the user and their family at any one time; who the key worker was, and when key workers changed.

- A sharing of skills and a celebration of people's work, which saw people developing skills which they almost certainly would not have done if they had remained in a uni-professional setting.

The chairing of the team was done on a rotational basis, and this was very useful in addressing some of the power issues between professions, and presenting a changed and more radical focus to the agencies concerned.

Professional supervision was undertaken through the professionals' lines of accountability.

We are taking relatively senior people in Health and Social Services and asking them to do something different. People have risen to the challenge and developed and enhanced their transferable skills.
            Director of Mental Health Services, from a
            background in clinical psychology.

In team working across disciplines, people sometimes forget the basics. John Adair's description of effective leadership as paying attention to three interlocking circles of mission or task, the team and individual needs, is sometimes lost sight of within the complexity of organisational concerns, (Adair, 1987 see Fig. 21, 194).

Cormack describes the needs that should be met for the team to achieve success as follows:

Mission or task:
- To set clear targets for the task.
- To set standards of performance.
- To make full use of resources.
- To clarify responsibilities.
- To ensure members' contributions are complementary.
- To achieve the set targets and standards.

Team needs:

- To know and respond to the leader's style and vision.
- To feel a common sense of purpose with members.
- To have a supportive climate.
- To grow and develop as a unit.
- To have a corporate sense of achievement.
- To have a common identity.

Individual needs (your own and others):

- To be accepted by the leader.
- To be valued by the leader.
- To be able to contribute to the task.
- To know what is expected in relation to the task.

- To be part of the team.
- To know what is expected of you by the team.

                                        Cormack, 1988.

To provide positive outcomes for people with mental health needs you have to connect primary care, secondary care and health and social care in a way so as they enhance each other.
        Director of Social Services and former Chief
                Executive of a Mental Health Trust.

The Sainsbury Centre's study of Community Mental Health Teams (Onyett, Pillinger and Muijen, 1995) shows a changing picture of CMHTs increasingly working as 'teams' in Payne's sense of the term, with team managers or co-ordinators, an organised and consistent referral system, shared record keeping etc. But at the time of the study, a large number were still operating as groups, for example, 53 per cent of the teams taking referrals via individual members rather than by a referral route which ensured that the team considered each referral with a team perspective.

The authors pay considerable 'attention to role ambiguity', because that 'is often cited as a source of stress and job dissatisfaction'. Putting:

Practitioners into teams places them in a special dilemma. They become members of two groups: their discipline and the team. As a result, they may find themselves torn between the aims of the Community Mental Health Movement that explicitly values egalitarianism, role blurring and a surrender of power to lower-status workers and service users on the one hand, and a desire to hold on to tradition, socially-valued role definitions and practices on the other.

The authors go on to say that:

*It might, therefore, be predicted that the ideal conditions for team membership would be where a positive sense of **belonging to the team can exist alongside continued professional identification.** This is most likely to occur when the discipline has a **clear and valued role within the team,** which in turn requires that the team itself has a clear role.*
            Onyett et al., 1995: p21–2 (my emphasis).

Who is going to keep my professional feet on the ground as I try and support people against the system?!
        social worker in a multi-disciplinary team.

The Sainsbury Study looks at the pressure on all the members of CMHT, and a great deal of those pressures do seem to be around role ambiguity and role changes, where individuals and groups have not been able to, or been allowed to, develop new ways of seeing themselves as valued. Psychiatrists, for example, appear to be 'vulnerable to burn out because they see themselves as having 'a lot of responsibility but not the corresponding authority'', (quoted in Onyett et al., 1995: p35).

The Study shows that 54 per cent of the social workers are:

Highly exhausted emotionally. Compared with other disciplines, they also have a comparatively low sense of personal accomplishment and a high degree of de-personalisation. They also have the least satisfaction with work relationships and least overall job satisfaction.

Onyett et al., 1995: p34.

The authors believe that this dissatisfaction may stem from:

- Confusion about their roles and their place in the team.
- Comparatively unclear about the role of the team and their focus within it.
- Low identification with their team and profession.
- Least positive sense of belonging to their profession.
- Confusion in regard to their roles as purchasers or providers of services (at the time of the study, community care and the care management role was relatively new. See also Macdonald and Sheldon's comments on the dichotomies of purchasing and providing).

The relationship between psychiatrist and social worker as both contribute to the care of people with mental health problems has shifted in various directions over the years, but it has always been an intimate one. In many ways, future Mental Health Services can be expected to be less dominated by a biomedical model as has been the case in recent years. All of the major developments: assertive outreach, home treatment, early intervention, etc. are around the development of different forms of psychosocial intervention.

consultant psychiatrist.

The social worker in primary care

Social workers have a specific contribution to make to the government's modernising agenda, with its emphasis on rights and responsibilities, citizenship and participation. Delivery of social care will be best offered in a collaborative approach from a range of professionals and agencies with the emphasis being around meeting the needs of individual consumers, their families and their communities.

GP with a regional and national role on mental health.

As we have seen from Chapter 1, the general practitioner is so often the first point of contact for individuals suffering from mental distress and their families. GPs recount a significant psychological component in 70 per cent of consultations, and in 20–25 per cent of patients a mental health problem will be their sole reason for consultation. As we have also noted, the interaction between physical and mental states of health and ill-health are profound, and it is the GP and members of the primary care team who are likely to be crucial in making a real difference for people who use their services.

Many of the issues around roles and team working, that have already been set out in the section on the Community Mental Health Team above, appertains to Primary Care Teams. Inevitably, resources in Social Services Departments are limited, and although some have made significant investments in attaching social workers to Primary Care Teams with great benefits (see Le Mesurier and Cumella's Study of Worcestershire, in *Managing Community Care*, 9: 1) but these social workers are normally targeted towards older persons and their families – including of course older people with a mental health need (either functional or organic). Studies, such as Le Mesurier and Cumella, demonstrate considerable benefits in preventing hospital admission and effecting speedier and effective discharge back to home or homely settings.

A model of innovative practice described by Firth et al. (2000) looks at five part-time and two full-time mental health workers attached to seven practices delivering services to patients/users referred directly by GPs. Of 200 referrals, only a dozen required assistance from secondary care services.

Social workers in primary care are also in a strategic position to affect partnership working and break down the silo mentality so as to ensure proper partnership in the service of users and carers.

The creation of the large and unified Health and Social Care Mental Health Trusts is producing a powerful and specialist focus for mental health services. One of the dangers is, however, that without clear leadership and an environmental perspective, they could become the children of the 19th century asylums, institutional and inward looking. It is absolutely essential that primary care drives the agenda as much as possible with a strong user, familial and social perspective, though this clearly has a

Case Example 9

Gambling on independence

A former social care manager is diagnosed with a disease that affects people with HIV and which severely impairs his cognitive ability. He develops mental health problems and is sectioned. A return to independence seems far off until social worker Paul Hatchman intervened.

Case notes

Practitioner: Paul Hatchman
Field: Social worker, health team (specialist HIV)
Location: London
Client: Richard Fraser (not his real name)
Case history: Just over two years ago, Fraser's health was deteriorating so badly that he was persuaded by friends to go to hospital. He was subsequently admitted and tests showed that he was HIV positive. Further tests showed that he had suspected progressive multifocal leukoencephalopathy (see Fact File, page 43), a disease associated with HIV that severely impairs cognitive ability. For example, Fraser became unable to wash himself, dress himself and so on. Survival is very rare, with death occurring usually between one and four months after contracting PML. He spent three months in an HIV specialist ward at a general hospital and was then admitted to a north London respite hospice. He was discharged home with an intensive 24-hour care package, but within a month began to display mental health difficulties that resulted in him being sectioned. He returned home only to be sectioned once again.
Dilemma: Fraser, an ex-social care manager, had difficulties in coming to terms with his illnesses, believing he could return to his usual way of life.
Risk factor: By increasing Fraser's independence, there is a danger that he might not manage his medication resulting in him being sectioned again.
Outcome: Fraser continues to improve and it is possible that future assessments might reduce his level of care further.

No longer considered newsworthy, you might be forgiven for thinking that HIV was no longer with us. But by the end of 2001 some 48,226 people in the UK had been diagnosed HIV positive, of which 3,342 were newly diagnosed that year. Since the introduction of combination therapy in 1996, death rates have dropped dramatically. More people (currently estimated at 33,000) are finding themselves able to live with HIV.

Life, however, was not something that Richard Fraser (not his real name)was thought to have much of left. Encouraged by his friends, who were alarmed at the deterioration of his health, he went to hospital and was subsequently diagnosed with HIV. Worse followed: he was also diagnosed with progressive multifocal leukoencephalopathy, a terminal and incurable illness that affects the nervous system.

PML usually takes between one and four months to claim its victims. It is very rare to survive this disease, but somehow Fraser did so. He was eventually discharged home, but with an intensive 24-hour care package.

Fraser, now 46, also developed mental health problems that resulted in him being sectioned twice. It was at this point that Paul Hatchman, social worker with the health (specialist HIV) team, became involved.

He immediately set about sorting out 'the nuts and bolts stuff', such as Fraser's housing benefit, disabled living allowance and professional pensions. It was clear that Fraser, an ex-social care manager, was in denial over his illness – possibly stemming from the shock of the dual diagnosis. 'He had come to terms with the HIV but not the PML. He wanted to go back to work. But I explained that wasn't realistic and he'd get angry and agitated. The pointers were all there, towards him getting violent and being sectioned again,' says Hatchman.

Hatchman supported Fraser through this traumatic period. 'I tried to understand where he was coming from,' he says. He was increasingly isolated, his circle of friends having faded away. 'We tried to address his aggression and convince him that we only wanted what was best for him. But he went through a stage when he wouldn't return calls or left rude messages.'

The other big challenge for Fraser was the loss of privacy that inevitably accompanies 24-hour care. 'There's only so much a carer can do and they'd sit with him and he'd just feel watched,' Hatchman says. He had four carers (all trainee doctors) who worked a rota. On occasion one would fail to turn up. What could have been a problem actually became an opportunity, as Fraser would manage to cope without a carer. 'After this had happened a few times we started to think about reducing the care hours,' says Hatchman. 'We agreed to take away the night care and that worked out fine.'

Further opportunities presented themselves: 'He'd call up and say that the carer hadn't turned up and he needed to go to the bank. So I'd say 'well, just go then'. And he would. So, slowly but surely he took on more independence.'

There have been times when Hatchman has 'sailed close to the wind' in his work with Fraser. Occasionally Fraser hasn't taken his anti-psychotic medication. 'He had worked in the drugs field and knows what these drugs can do to your head, so he wouldn't take them. But he'd become aggressive.' His carers had informally monitored his medication, but with their reduced hours this was no longer possible.

However, Fraser has managed his medication well. The community psychiatric nurse visits fortnightly now rather than daily. He even attends courses at the London Lighthouse, studying for a teaching qualification. Although he is aware that he may never teach, the personal esteem and confidence this promotes is immeasurable.

Fraser's continual improvement, mentally and physically, has meant that he now has just two care hours in the morning and three in the evening. And this may even be reduced further. Hatchman says that Fraser recently facilitated a group at the Lighthouse on HIV and drugs awareness: 'I went along and there were about five other professionals there as well. And apart from me, no one knew about his status. I was very impressed and the feedback was very positive.'

Hatchman's work with Fraser highlights the positive support that can help bring some normality back to a life shattered by HIV and, most impressively, PML. 'I compare him now with those times when he has been very low, depressed, confused and disorientated. And he is such a different man.' And quite a remarkable one, too.

Arguments for risk

- Fraser's physical health was improving and it was reasonable to build on this and encourage more independence. The more that he was able to do things for himself the more his confidence and self-esteem would improve, thereby positively affecting his mental health.
- Clearly the more independent Fraser is, the better his quality of life. By moving, however gradually, to developing his independence, it would go some way to combating the trauma of the double diagnosis of HIV and PML and restore some normality back to his life.
- The isolation suffered through his condition and loss of work and friends needed to be tackled, or else there would be a real danger that Fraser might deteriorate further. Attempts to introduce social contacts may help to reduce Fraser's helplessness and, in turn, his frustration and aggression.
- Fraser had demonstrated that on occasion he could manage with reduced care, and he was willing to try and do more for himself.

Arguments against risk

- Fraser had not always managed his medication well -either forgetting or deliberately refusing to take it (on one occasion his carers found a small number of tablets tucked away in his pockets).

The removal of full-time care meant that the informal monitoring of his medication by his carers would be lost – adding to the risk.

- Should he not take his anti-psychotic medication, his subsequent aggressive behaviour may be misinterpreted, resulting in him being possibly sectioned.
- Should he not take his HIV medication there would be a strong possibility that he would build up a resistance to it. This may lead to the further possibility that he may run out of effective medicines to stabilise his health. The side-effects can also be quite harmful.
- There is always the possibility that if things were not working out and he believed he would never have his old life back, he might at best deteriorate further, or worse take his own life.

Independent comment

Fraser faced the complexity of an HIV positive diagnosis and possible deteriorating cognitive impairment at a time when his physical health was severely affected, writes Grainne Morby. Any diagnosis of a potentially life threatening condition, particularly HIV with its associated stigma, has a damaging effect on self-esteem.

Fraser was provided 24-hour medical care package by four different people, which also helped combat perceived risks such as self-harm and non-adherence to treatments. He, however, believed it was over-controlling and did not welcome it.

Breakdowns in the care package led to an increased emphasis on supporting Fraser's independence which, with the peer support and personal development opportunities, suggests that he is learning to live independently with HIV. It is very likely though that, without Paul's encouragement and practical support on diagnosis, the positive outcome would have been less certain.

A person is better equipped to deal with the consequences both of their HIV diagnosis and the knock-on effect it will have on the rest of their life if health and social care are combined early enough after diagnoses of HIV.

Terrence Higgins Trust and Lighthouse are in the process of establishing a social care centre. This will enable people living with HIV to receive both medical and social care support, and reflects the growing need for a more holistic approach to the delivery of care packages.

Grainne Morby is director of London services at the Terrence Higgins Trust.

Reprinted by kind permission of *Community Care*, 7–13 March, 2002.

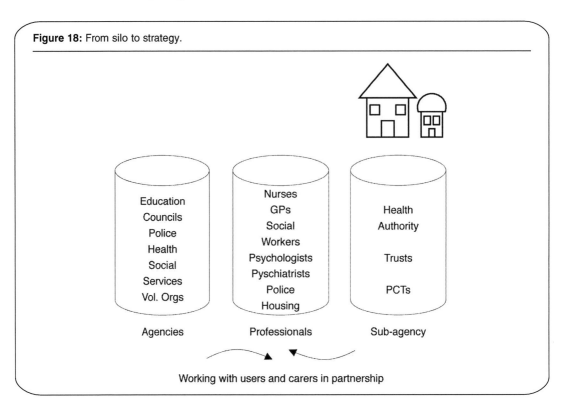

Figure 18: From silo to strategy.

Education
Councils
Police
Health
Social
Services
Vol. Orgs

Nurses
GPs
Social
Workers
Psychologists
Pyschiatrists
Police
Housing

Health
Authority

Trusts

PCTs

Agencies   Professionals   Sub-agency

Working with users and carers in partnership

lot of issues about strengthening mental health commissioning within primary care trusts and ensuring that they are really reflecting community needs in the way that primary care groups had begun to do before their demise (see Behan and Loft, 1999).

The really effective primary care team is invaluable in promoting sound mental health. As one general practitioner puts it:

> *Most patients present their problems as undifferentiated mixtures of physical, emotional, family and social symptoms. And yet we organise whole systems of health and social care, which separate the biomedical from the psychological and social. The limitation of such a simplistic 'body and mind' approach is challenged by several studies of mental disorders in primary care which consistently report the co-occurrence of physical, emotional and social problems in patients, and furthermore show such patients to be the highest utilisers of these services* (see Barrett et al., 1988; Bridges and Goldberg, 1985; Kaplan et al., 1988; Katon et al., 1992; Katon et al., 1990).
>
> General practitioner with a policy role.

Conclusion

With society and family life increasingly fragmented and under a range of pressures, the need for skilled helpers to consider the needs and aspirations of individuals within their family, community and social context, is even more acute now than when social work first began to put down roots in the middle of the 19th century. In times of crisis, or when life becomes a long and bitter struggle for survival, then people in distress turn to someone who is genuine, who listens, hears, and who produces practical results.

Chapter 6

The Vital Equilibrium – The Role of the Approved Social Worker

These unhappy persons are outcasts from all the social and domestic affections of private life . . . and have no refuge but in the law. You can prevent, by the agency which you shall appoint as you have in so many incidences prevented, the occurrence of frightful cruelty; you can soothe . . . and restore many sufferers to health and usefulness . . .

Lord Ashley, (later the 7th Earl of Shaftesbury), Houses of Parliament, 23rd July 1844.

The ASW's role is therefore complex and, at times, beset with problems of both practice and principle. However, we continue to believe that ASWs play a vital role in the administration of the Act. If an equivalent role in new legislation is to be undertaken by a wider professional group . . . we urge the Government to consider how the benefits of the current structure might be protected.

The Mental Health Act Commission, 9th Biennial Report, 1999–2001, para. 2.48, p15.

The role of the social worker in mental health is to operate on the margin . . . The ASW is freed up to act in the best interests of the service user and to apply the guidance contained within the Act and the code of practice. This unusual level of autonomy is pivotal to the role, which was intended to provide a failsafe against inappropriate use of the powers of detention. A counterbalance to the draconian powers which can allow the removal of liberty without the scrutiny of the Courts.

practising approved social worker.

ASW training is gold standard.

Judy Foster, responsible for mental health issues, TOPSS.

Social workers have traditionally been and continue to be concerned with enabling people to have control over their lives, promoting people's rights of citizenship and protecting those who are at risk in the least restrictive way . . . social workers occupy a unique statutory role . . . it is of critical importance that at least one professional application maintains some independence from the others.

from response by Northamptonshire Approved Social Workers Standards Group to proposals for reform of the Mental Health Act, 1983.

What is liberty and how can it best be safeguarded? All societies have these problems. How they answer them depends on what they are and the values they hold.

Kathleen Jones, 1972: pxiii.

English common law – the lay perspective

The recent radio broadcast, in June 2002, of dialogue from the Putney Debates which took place at the end of the British Civil War, and the historical/legal commentary which accompanied the Radio 4 programme, highlights how much British society today is a result of dialogue, opinion forming, power bloc pressure, conflict (armed or not) and legal ebb and flow over many years.

British political and social life is often a search for some form of consensus and equilibrium between conflicting, sometimes violently conflicting, views and interests. While usually the scales of law and implements are weighted in favour of the powerful, still there are countervailing influences, both ethical and pragmatic, which shape the state of society we live in and the attitudes of those who govern. Naked power can never be enough either in organisational governance or in constitutional governance. King Alfred of Wessex and England was given his sobriquet 'The Great', because his conception of kingship, stemming from a Judaic-Christian formulation and his close identification with the people because of the external threat of the Danish invasions, created an amazing synthesis between authority, legislation, and the practice of governance (see e.g. Wallace-Hadrill, 1971). It was partly Charles the First's inability or unwillingness to recognise that leaders, to a great extent, rely on those they purport to lead which led to the Civil War.

The Putney Debates, and so much of what has taken place as political discourse right up to the present day in Britain, is about the nature of government and authority and who should wield that authority in what circumstances.

Into this debate comes the nature of the laws which stem from social policy and lead on to social practice (see Jenkins, McCulloch, Friedli and Parker, 2002; Jenkins, 2001; Jones, 1972; Hoggett, 1984; Olsen, 1984; Brayne and Martin, 1999).

A number of themes which are most important in the context of the role of the approved social worker under mental health legislation are:

- The separation of powers – executive and legislative.
- Issues around liberty and safety.
- The need for constitutional checks and balances.

In the recent review of tribunals, Sir Andrew Leggatt remarks in his overview:

> Most importantly, they (the tribunals) are not independent of the departments that sponsor them. The object of this review is to recommend a system that is **independent**, coherent, professional, cost-effective and user-friendly.
>
> Leggatt, March 2001: p5 (my emphasis).

In mental health law particularly, where the liberty of the individual is at risk (both physical and psychological liberty) such liberty of the individual has to be balanced against their safety and that of other people – as the Mental Health Act 1983 states 'He [sic] ought to be so detained in the interests of his own health or safety or with a view to the protection of other persons', (Mental Health Act, 1983: Section 2 (2) (b)).

In this it is most important to maintain a philosophical perspective. Whether one believes with Spinoza that 'the true aim of government is liberty', (*Ethics*, 1677) or with his near contemporary Hobbes, that humankind's greatest fear is social chaos, the history of mental health law, policy and practice shows society as a whole and practitioners in particular grappling with the concepts and the practicalities of weighing freedom before the law with a need to protect individuals from the extreme consequences of their own and others' actions. In essence, we still work on the lines laid down by John Stuart Mill that:

> The sole end for which mankind are warranted, individually or collectively, in interfering with the liberty of action of any of their number, is self-protection.
>
> On Liberty, 1859.

But these general propositions while vital foundations and guides, do not provide the whole story for the doctor, social worker, police officer, CPN, at 2 a.m. Nevertheless, it is philosophy and the development of legislation which gives such a strong impetus to the need for a check and balance to the dominant professional viewpoint at any one time in history. At the present time, it is the approved social worker, employed by local authorities. This role has a long provenance (see Table 5 below), but it is worth quoting the Percy Commission (1957), who were charged with evaluating mental health legislation and making proposals, which led to the 1959 Mental Health Act. Brenda Hoggett quotes the Commission as recording that:

Although 'no responsible relative or mental welfare officer would likely disregard or dissent from the doctor's advice', the report was clear that they must be free to do so', (quoted in Hoggett, 1984: p74).

In essence, the approved social worker is:

- A vital check and balance in the evaluation of whether someone needs compulsory admission to hospital.
- The provider of specialist assessment skills, with a humanistic/holistic/social/familial/environmental and systems perspective.
- A knowledge-bearer and co-ordinator of resources so as to provide the least restricted alternative for the service user.

Stanley and Manthorpe, in their work on the Mental Health Enquiries, identify:

> The unique role of the ASW as the co-ordinator of assessments, a repository of legal and procedural knowledge and the representative of the link with other areas of Social Services and local authority provision. Social work can also offer a broader social and family perspective to assessment and care planning as well as experience in communication and support for carers and the potential for applying skills in family interventions. In the context of the relationship with individual service users, social work represents a holistic, humanistic approach with an established commitment to anti-oppressive practice.
>
> Stanley and Manthorpe, 2001: p96.

Margaret Clayton, chairperson of the Mental Health Act Commission, in a recent article has a clear message from the visitations that the MHAC has made during 1999 to 2001 '. . . the role of the Approved Social Worker (ASW) in the care of patients with acute mental illness is crucial'. (Clayton, 2002: p38).

Because it is sometimes asserted that social workers are only concerned with liberty and not with safety, it is worth considering the independent enquiry into the care and treatment afforded to Benjamin Rathbone (Mackay et al., November 2001). On the 18th February 1999, Benjamin Rathbone attacked a

Table 5: The evolution of the approved social worker.

Date	Case worker	Authorised officer
1834 Poor Law Act		Poor law relieving officer
1913 Mental Deficiency Act	Mental deficiency visitor	Poor law relieving officer, some acting as 'specially authorised officer'
1929 Local Government Act and 1930 Mental Treatment Act	Mental deficiency visitors and psychiatric social workers	Public assistance officers acting as 'duly authorised officers'
1948 Implementation of National Health Service Act	Mental Health social workers	As above
1954 Formation of Society of Mental Welfare Officers	'Mental welfare officers'	
1959 Mental Health Act	Mental Welfare Officers (created by statute)	
1971 Implementation of Local Authority Social Services Act	Social workers	Social workers (operating as MWOs for the purposes of the 1959 Act)
1974 National Health Service Re-organisation	Hospital social workers became part of social services	
1983 Mental Health Act	Generic and specialist social workers	Approved Social Workers

Gilbert, 1985: p61.

man on Loughborough station and pushed him into the path of an oncoming train. Amazingly, the victim survived.

In June 1999, the sentencing judge pronounced to Rathbone 'It's quite plain that you are suffering from mental illness'. An enquiry was set up to evaluate the events and found:

- Poor self-awareness from Rathbone and limited compliance with the prescribed treatment.
- Poor follow-up by the CMHT into the community.
- An over reliance on feedback from Benjamin's father.
- A repeat pattern of leave from hospital without realistic evaluation of the situation.
- Risk assessments undertaken but not appropriately acted on.

The role of the social worker was specifically praised by the enquiry team. He provided the essential interlinking element and relationship between Rathbone, his family and other members of the team, and was clearly balancing issues of liberty and safety in a realistic manner. Unfortunately, the case was closed to social services and the leadership/management problems within the team prevented proper appropriate action to be taken of the social work assessments.

In October 1998, the social worker undertook a risk assessment and indicated the following risk factors:

- Poor compliance with medication.
- Clear evidence of the risk of violence to others on becoming unwell.
- A risk to himself, especially in view of his suicide attempt.
- Poor therapeutic relationships with the professionals involved in his case.
- Misuse of alcohol and drugs.
- Continual denial of past and current illness leading to lack of engagement.

The enquiry team praised the social worker for:

- A thorough process and good written records.
- 'A very comprehensive risk assessment', a comment made by the Consultant Psychiatrist.
- The maintaining of a relationship with Benjamin Rathbone, though as the social worker himself said: 'I don't think I had anything special, but I did find that if you just stuck with him and kept coming back at it, he was somebody that you got glimmers of engagement, which were quite important'.
- A positive relationship with the carers, who perceived that Benjamin revealed more to the social worker than anyone else.
- An appreciation of the family and social context. As the enquiry report comments on

Table 6: Historical path of legislation and committal.

Legislation	Ethos of the legislation	Typology of user	Typology of Admission	Section of Act	Responsible officers designated
1744 Vagrancy Act.	Containment.	'Lunatic or mad person'.	Detention, restraint, maintenance and curing.		2 or more Justices
1808 County Asylum Act.		Persons dangerous to be at large.		17–19	On a warrant from 2 Justices
NB 'Criminal lunatics' dealt with somewhat separately under the Criminal Lunatics Act 1800.					
1845 Lunatics Act.	Care. The Institution as therapeutic.	(i) Private. Insane, idiot, of unsound mind. (ii) Pauper.			Petitioner (relative) plus 2 separate medical practitioners. Petitioner (relative or other), JP or clergyman of the parish plus relieving officer or overseer
1890 Lunacy Act.	'The triumph of legalism' (Kathleen Jones). Protecting the individual against inappropriate confinement.	Private	Reception Order	4–8	Petitioner (relative or other), statement before a JP supported by 2 medical certificates.
		Pauper.	Urgency Order	11	Petitioner plus 1 medical certificate.
			Summary Reception Order.	13–22	Poor Law relieving officer or police make application to JP. One medical certificate required
1930 Mental Treatment Act.	Accent on treatment and maintaining 'social equilibrium' (Royal Commission). Introduction of voluntary admission.	Certified patient			As under 1890 Act
		Temporary patient			Nearest relative plus 2 medical certificates
		Voluntary.			N/A
1959 Mental Health Act.	Optimism in medical treatment. Community approaches. Informal admission.	Admission for observation.		25	2 medical practitioners
		Admission for treatment		26	2 medical practitioners – usually GP and specialist. Mental welfare officer or nearest relative
		Emergency admission.		29	Application from mental welfare officer or nearest relative plus one medical practitioner

	Admission for assessment	2	Application by ASW/nearest relative 2 medical practitioners
	Admission for treatment.	3	As above
	Admission for assessment in cases of emergency.	4	ASW/nearest relative 1 medical practitioner
1983 Mental Health Act.	Pendulum swings back to legal ethos Protection of civil rights. Some scepticism over the efficacy of treatment programmes and whether community care was rhetoric or reality.		
2003 Mental Health Act?	Greater confidence in efficacy of treatment. Increase in evidence-based care and treatment options. Increased concern over public safety		
2025 Mental Health Act?	Resurfacing of anxieties over consent, compulsion and civil rights?		

the fact that Social Services closed the case: 'However, as subsequently evolved, the Social Work skills of relationship development and of working with the social network would have added value to that role'. The enquiry team clearly felt it important to stress that the *role* of the social worker as well as the specific skills of the individual worker were an important component of a team approach with somebody of Benjamin Rathbone's character and history, (Mackay, 2001: p20).

The developing role of the social worker

To recognise the importance of the approved social worker role, it is necessary to take a historical perspective. In 18th century England, there was considerable fear of the mobile poor (described as vagrants) and people suffering from a mental disorder. The practical tolerance of the mediaeval monasteries and the philosophical toleration of writers such as the physician Paracelsus had vanished under the pressures of social dislocation; agrarian reform and industrialisation; paranoia around social chaos and social mobility since the Civil War; and particular fears amongst the propertied classes.

The spirit of the age is often expressed in the context of art and architecture. In Shakespeare's *King Lear*, the rational are destroyed by their pragmatism, while a 'fool' and a 'madman' lead 'aged folly' and 'blindness' to sanity and salvation. Disease and disorder in its various forms were acknowledged and in some ways appreciated. The radical William Erbery went so far as to say:

> *If madness be the heart of man, Ecclesiastes verse 9, chapter 3, then this is the island of Great Bedlam, come let us all be mad together.*
> The Madman's Plea, quoted in Hill, 1975.

The Restoration following the Civil War, and the advent of the Classical Age, presaged an era during which the forces of nature are thrown back. The gates at the great classical palaces, such as Versailles and Blenheim, are in the form of twisted thorny barbs, guarding the building and courtyard from the great park, which itself keeps untamed nature at bay. The Classical Age is in all senses the time when the gates are closed and reason shielded from folly. When the hospital of Bethlem was burned down, it was rebuilt on the model of a French palace; the great American asylums, such as Pennsylvania, are modelled on a pattern of European palaces.

The Classical Age is essentially agoraphobic, even on the stage when we have moved from the wildness of Shakespeare's *A Midsummer Night's Dream*, to the stately pageant of Purcell's *Fairy Queen*.

After the ferment of 1649–60, it is perhaps not surprising that Hobbes's appeal to the 'reasonable' side of man found so large a response, that madness which had been the garment of many political radicals should be mistrusted, and that the enclosure of marginal lands and marginal men should be vigorously applied.

In the first half of the 18th century, people suffering from a mental illness could be confined as follows:

- Those confined under the Poor Laws – the responsibility of the parish overseer.
- Those confined under the criminal law – until 1800 insanity was not an effective defence against a criminal charge.
- Those confined under the vagrancy laws – those considered vagrants were harshly dealt with.
- Those confined in private madhouses. These were run for profit. The only defence against confinement was by means of a writ of Habeas Corpus, but the secrecy and restraint used by the owners of these institutions made it very difficult to make such appeal.
- Patients in Bethlem – financed by public subscriptions and legacies.
- 'Single lunatics' – usually confined and cared for at home, e.g. Mrs. Rochester in Charlotte Bronte's *Jane Eyre*.

see Jones, 1972: Ch. 1.

As we can see from Table 6, matters progressed but often in a series of circles, not in a straight line. The 1744 Vagrancy Act began to see more distinction between vagrants and those suffering from a mental disorder. It also introduced a form of check and balance in that two or more Justices had to be brought into play to confine somebody suffering from a mental illness, whereas a vagrant merited only a single Magistrate's warrant. No medical opinion was deemed necessary and as the belief was that mental illness was one distinct state differing so markedly from ordinary mental health, and easily identifiable, as well as being a continuous state, it was very difficult for individuals to prove that they had recovered.

Private madhouses came under scrutiny in the 1760s when instances were discovered of persons being placed there by relatives for sinister reasons. Wives who had become inconvenient, elderly relations, whose money was coveted, were extremely vulnerable, and the genesis of regulation can be seen in the passing of the 1774 Act to Licence and Regulate the Private Madhouse. Issues such as licensing, notification of reception of people considered mentally disordered, visitation by commissioners, inspection and supervision by the medical profession, look ahead to the regulatory framework of the 21st century.

Although attitudes towards people with a mental illness gradually became more positive during the latter part of the 18th and early 19th centuries, partly perhaps due to sympathy for George III in his severe bouts of mental distress, it took the passionate championing and legislative muscle of Lord Ashley (later the 7th Earl of Shaftesbury) to make a real and lasting difference to both public attitudes and practical care. Shaftesbury's leadership is a shining example because he always saw the conditions of the poor, deprived, distressed and dispossessed for himself before proposing action, and he was driven not only by his profound religious beliefs but an awareness of his own tendency to severe bouts of depression, and an unhappy childhood.

The Lunatics Act of 1845 had as its predominant principle the need to ensure that those suffering from a mental illness received care and treatment as soon as possible.

Kathleen Jones writes:

After the passing of the 1845 Act, there were three possible channels for further reform. It could develop along the social and humanitarian lines laid down at the Retreat ... it could develop along purely medical lines, blurring the distinction between mental and physical disorders, sharing in the great developments which characterised general medicine in the second half of the 19th century; or it could proceed along legal lines, piling safeguard on safeguard to protect the sane against illegal detention. In the social approach, the emphasis was on human relations; in the medical approach, it was on physical treatment, in the legal approach, it was on procedure.

Jones, K., 1972: p153.

Perhaps inevitably the pendulum swung towards concerns over liberty, reinforced by a number of cause célèbres, and leading to the Lunacy Act of 1890 which Jones terms 'the triumph of legalism'.

The 20th century began to see the pendulum turn back more towards treatment and also

Case Example 10

'Jack Williamson' was a man of white English heritage in his mid-thirties, and the ASW received a referral from the local consultant psychiatrist, for an assessment under the Mental Health Act, after the latter had spoken with Mr Williamson and decided that the parents were no longer able to continue caring for Jack because of his current mental ill-health. The social worker instigated an assessment and liaised with Jack's GP, who agreed to attend, and also with ambulance staff and police because it was anticipated that there could be difficulties in conveying Jack to hospital, should compulsory admission be deemed necessary.

Unfortunately, the initial assessment had to be aborted as the consultant psychiatrist was not able to attend for reasons beyond anybody's control, and Jack drove off.

The social worker spent some time with Jack's parents, both to ascertain more information regarding the circumstances surrounding care for Jack, and also to assess risk. He then liaised again with the police over risk elements.

Some days later, the police got in touch with the social worker to say that they had arrested Jack for an assault on a member of the public.

The aborted assessment visit created a number of subsequent problems, which the ASW had to deal with. Jack's parents were torn between feeling that they were unable to continue caring for Jack at present because of the state of his health and also because they were frightened of him. At the same time, they seemed to underestimate the risk that Jack posed to other people, and they were ambivalent about working with statutory services. The 'Williamsons' were an articulate, middle class family, and Mr Williamson had an official position in the community which tended to over-influence some sections of the statutory services.

Subsequent to Jack's arrest, an assessment was carried out by the ASW and two doctors. Jack was admitted to a semi-secure unit based on the risk he posed to members of the public.

There were differences of opinion in terms of the level of risk posed, and the ASW's appreciation of the whole picture was essential to ensure the correct placement to suit Jack's needs and those of other people. The ASW's intervention was crucial also to repairing relationships between the family and the statutory services, and assisting them in looking forward realistically to taking up the caring role again, when Jack was discharged.

The ASW recorded the learning points in respect of the ASW competencies set down by the educational body:

- The application of the values of social work – balancing the risk with Jack's rights in respect of the assessment process. Placing Jack in the context of his needs and both past and present behaviour, working with him in the context of a relationship through the statutory process and beyond into discharge and the future.
- Exercising the duties, powers and responsibilities of an ASW – undertaking the lead in the assessment, and ensuring that issues around individual rights and the law were maintained.
- Making informed decisions – making decisions in the light of all the circumstances.
- Working to identify, influence and use networks and collaborative arrangements – this was especially crucial following the abortive first assessment, and the need to liaise effectively with a number of statutory agencies.
- Working effectively in complex situations. The relationships within the family and between the family and statutory services could have placed Jack, his family and/or the public in a very difficult position. The ASW unscrambled these competing issues and perspectives.

social perspectives and approaches, with the renovated and reformed local authorities being asked to take on additional responsibilities for community services. The 1959 Mental Health Act was born out of an optimism in the efficacy of the new drugs regimes, and a belief that community alternatives to hospitals would invariably proliferate. Olsen, however, points out that the 1959 Act sacrificed a number of legal safeguards. Prior to 1959:

> . . . *except in instances where a person was wandering at large, a Duly Authorised Officer was required to make a statement before a Justice before effecting a compulsory admission to hospital. This requirement had the benefit of providing some defence of the patient's rights, ensuring the propriety of the admission, and guarding against wrongful certification . . . The Mental Health Act 1959 reflected the optimism generated by new drugs, new skills, changing attitudes, and a developing social service, and abolished the Justice's involvement in the procedure.*
> Olsen, 1984: p17.

In reality, the statements around community care were more rhetoric than reality. While some health authorities attempted to handle the hospital and reprovision programme in an ethical manner, transferring resources to new community services (health, social services, independent sector), others were seduced by the idea of appropriating the money for other purposes. I well remember going to an official seminar by a then Regional Health Authority whose approach to hospital reprovision was a quite explicit urging of everybody 'to find the financial loophole' in social security systems and use them so that money locked up in the institutions could be siphoned off for use elsewhere. As I was at the time attempting to find people lost in the system by the Health Service and a London borough that I was working with at the time, and finding them poorly supported in dubious private residential care run nakedly for profit, the seminar was one of the most disillusioning I have ever attended!

As Richard Titmuss remarked with some acerbity:

> *If English social history is any guide, confusion has often been the mother of complacency . . . what some hope will exist is suddenly thought by many to exist.*
> Titmuss, 1961, quoted in Jones, K. 1988: p33.

The 1983 Mental Health Act was partly framed in an atmosphere of disillusionment with 'Care in the Community' as a concept. The House of Commons Social Services Committee was to remark two years after the passing of the Act that the phrase had become 'virtually meaningless . . . it has become a slogan, with all the weakness that implies', (HCSS, 1985: para. 8). It pointed out the way in which the phrase had been used e.g.

- Saving money on the present costs of hospital care by getting people out of hospital, but not necessarily into proper alternative care.
- The transfer of responsibility from the NHS to local authorities.
- The transfer of care from statutory services to families and volunteers.

At the same time the Committee was indicating the 'large numbers' 'sleeping rough and under railway bridges, some within hailing distance of the Palace of Westminster', (HCSS, 1985: para. 162). Studies in America by Andrew Scull were revealing that rapid transfer of responsibilities, changes in funding mechanisms and reduced regulation were leading to the creation of what Michael Dear and Jennifer Wolch termed *'landscapes of despair'*, (homelessness and destitution), and *'The landscape of haunted places'* (the re-creation of the Institution) (Dear and Wolch, 1987).

In all this time, the mental welfare officer was having to work against the background of an act which had been framed in optimism, and attempting to balance issues of liberty, safety and appropriate treatment. Richard Jones in his seventh edition of the *Mental Health Act Manual*, (Jones, R., 2001) quotes Lord Justice Devlin as stating that:

> *It is the business of the duly authorised officer, rather than that of the doctor, to see that statutory powers are not used for the purpose (of hospital treatment) unless the circumstances warrant it.*
> Buxton v. Jayne, 1960; Jones, R. 2001: p86.

The 1983 Mental Health Act

Kathleen Jones, who favours the social and treatment approaches above the legal, sees the Mental Health Act 1959 as 'an enabling Act', while in her view 'the new law marked a return to legalism'. Jones sees the 1983 Mental Health Act as a return to the concerns of 1890, 'a prescriptive Act', making sure that different professions followed specific procedures. 'In its final form, it represented an uneasy compromise between the civil rights concerns of MIND and what the DHSS lawyers thought it possible to achieve by law', (Jones, K., 1988: p39).

Furthermore, Jones sees the Act as focusing on a very small number of people, not really touching the issues for the majority of people in hospital and the much greater numbers in community settings. Olsen, in his historical analysis of the key factors which led to the amendment of the Mental Health Act of 1959, points to community care still being 'simply a statement of objectives', in the words of the then Secretary of State for Social Services, Barbara Castle, (Olsen, 1984: p14, quoting DHSS, 1975). While policy was becoming increasingly community focused, with 95 per cent of all people with mental illness living in the community in the late 1970s, only 5 per cent of the overall mental health budget was devoted to their needs. Olsen, who as an academic, was also in touch with many practice areas at the time, also expressed concern that the apparent solution to emergency situations was to remove the individual to hospital 'no matter whether the cause is thought to lie within the person himself, the nature of his relationships, the social environment, or in disease processes', (Olsen op. cit. p15–6). Olsen criticised the lack of teamwork between professions, the limited understanding of respective roles and obligations and the co-ordination of the admission process.

Olsen also makes a very telling point about the role of what one might call 'the balancing agent' in the admissions process, and how optimism regarding the growth in treatment and service options may lead us to a false optimism around the need to consider the checks and balances when issues of individual liberty are involved. Olsen's comments regarding the role of the checks and balances involved in admission are highly relevant to the debate which is now under way in the reform of the 1983 Act, with the launch of the draft Mental Health Bill (DoH, 2002: Cmd. 5538-1, and its accompanying explanatory notes and issues for consultation):

The Mental Health Act 1959 reflected the optimism generated by new drugs, new skills, changing attitudes and the developing social services, and abolished the justice's involvement in the procedure. However, in so doing, it did not clearly prescribe who should take over the Justice's specific responsibilities, and many thought that the MWO would assume this role. This was not to be. The ambiguity of the 1959 Act, the weakness of the social worker's position relative to the power of the alliance between GP and psychiatrist . . . ensured that this role would not be assumed by the social worker or
anyone else party to the procedure. **The result was that the safeguards previously offered to the patient were lost***.*

> Olsen, op. cit. p17 (my emphasis).

The more I consider the issue, the more I believe that the loss of the specific ASW role under the proposals for the new Act, the possible diminution of a social perspective and the appointment of approved mental health professionals within the same agency framework as the psychiatrists, will in fact create both real and perceived problems around the compulsory orders which will undermine other positive aspects of the proposals.

Reform of the 1983 Mental Health Act

For reasons already discussed, the 1983 Act began to be seen in the 1990s as an interim piece of legislation and the Government established an independent expert review committee under the chairmanship of Professor Genevra Richardson which reported in November 1999. The following year, the government published a white paper on the need for reform to mental health legislation (Reforming the Mental Health Act, Cmd. 5016). The main impetus for legislation from the government point of view was to:

- Bring legislation into line with current practice, recognising that in Mental Health as in other service areas (child care, intermediate care, in work with older people, strategies and practice in learning disability services, etc.) the balance needed to shift to viewing the system as a whole rather than concentrating on acute hospital care.
- Bringing the law into line with the European Convention on Human Rights, especially following the enactment of the Human Rights Act, 1998 in England in 2000 (See Sainsbury Centre briefing on the Human Rights Act – Briefing No. 12).
- Removing the 'treatability' clause as there was a danger of a number of people who were not so much untreatable as difficult to treat being denied a service.

I will not go into all of the issues around the proposed reforms of the Mental Health Act here, as an excellent briefing is contained in the Sainsbury Centre Briefing No. 14 (March 2001). It is worth remarking, however, that the press coverage on the 26th June 2002, following the debate in the House of Commons the previous day, focused in on issues around Community Treatment Orders and issues around the detention of people with dangerous and severe personality disorder (DSPD). Part of the dilemma facing the Government is the confusion that clearly exists in the public mind between the needs and potential dangerousness of people with severe personality disorders, and those with a treatable mental illness.

The Times headline on the 26th June was: 'Dangerous psychopaths may be held indefinitely', (p10).

Case Example 11

Section 136 of the 1983 Mental Health Act empowers a police constable to remove an individual from a public place if they 'think it necessary to do so in the interests of that person or for the protection of other persons' and the individual can be detained for a period not exceeding 72 hours for the purpose of having them examined by a registered medical practitioner and to be interviewed by an approved social worker. The existence of trained, experienced and skilled individuals with a social work perspective has enabled a number of people at risk to be assessed in a way which has then avoided compulsory admission to hospital.

One practitioner recalls interviewing a young man who seemed extremely confused. The psychiatrist was keen to admit, but the social worker was convinced that there was another issue here. In the end, she discovered that the medication he was on for the treatment of leukaemia had had an adverse reaction, and she was able to gain physical treatment for him and avoid admission.

A second very similar case involved a woman with diabetes, who had become so confused through the reduction of her blood sugar levels, that she was completely incoherent. The social worker's intuition was that for whatever reason, she needed nutriment, and gradually, as she was fed, the woman's confusion and agitation ceased and she became lucid, and was able to return home.

In a third instance, an individual with a tendency to depression combined alcohol with medication and became aggressive. Approached by the police, the individual became violent and was taken to a place of safety – in this instance a room in a hospital, not a police station (an arrangement between the local NHS Trust and the Police Service). Again, the ASW felt that there were other factors involved than a specific mental illness, and was clear to both the police and the nursing staff that she couldn't properly assess the individual in this condition. After a couple of hours, the toxic reaction wore off, and the person concerned was very grateful to the social worker for avoiding compulsory admission.

The social worker had to work through the anxieties of the hospital staff and police.

In my own experience, I recall being called out to a police station at 2 a.m. The police had found a woman wandering around the shops in the early morning, and were not sure what her mental state was, and as she would not communicate with them, and had no obvious means of identification, they were nonplussed. When I sat down with her with a cup of tea, my instinct was that she might have a mild learning disability and so I used Makaton sign language while I was verbally communicating with her. Immediately I used sign language, she commenced speaking. My supposition would be that as soon as she saw the sign language, she recognised somebody who might be helpful to her in line with staff that she knew who used that means of communication. As soon as she started speaking, it was relatively easy to elicit that she lived in supported housing in Brighton, and had got confused and frightened and disorientated on a shopping expedition to Burgess Hill. I was able to liaise with her support workers and return her to her home.

The *Independent*'s headline was: 'Anger at plan for indefinite detention of people with dangerous mental disorders', (p4).

Both papers have photographs of Michael Stone (diagnosed with a personality disorder), who murdered Lynne and Megan Russell, and Christopher Clunis (diagnosed as schizophrenic) who killed Jonathan Zito.

Despite a growing public awareness that we are all vulnerable to mental ill-health, it is clear that the 'moral panic' is still alive and well. The well-intentioned concept of expanding compulsion into community settings, and at the same time tackling issues around dangerous and severe personality disorder, may make it very difficult to gain the right balance between liberty and safety. For mental health legislation and practice to work, then there has to be the correct balance between the two. Health Minister, Jacqui Smith, in her speech made it clear that most people with mental health problems were not a risk to themselves or others, but that the Government had a duty to protect those that were and the public. If the balance between care, treatment, liberty, safety for individuals and the public are not kept in a state of equilibrium, then we will simply see another build up of the pressure through moral panics and the whole cycle start again.

On the 29th June this year, concern was expressed in the media concerning the release from secure hospital into a community hospital of Eden Strang, who less than three years ago had attacked a church congregation in London with a Samurai sword. The comments from the church where the attack had occurred spoke of fear, concern for the perpetrator, concern for the victims, and a desire to forgive and not to exclude, but at the same time to ensure that Eden Strang remained healthy and would no longer pose a danger to others. The comments were very supportive of a legislative framework which would ensure that the capacity for compulsion could overarch the hospital and community settings so as to ensure that the treatment necessary to ensure a healthy life and safety should be available to the individual without withdrawal or some form of administrative break.

Most people might feel it was appropriate to detain someone like Michael in hospital – but in Bradford I saw a different way of dealing with a similar patient. Matthew had smashed the doors of a health centre, harassed shoppers and recently had thrown a road sign at a woman parking her car (it didn't hit her). Instead of bringing him into hospital under Section, a psychiatrist and a social worker went out to find Matthew on the streets and spent half an hour negotiating with him, with 40 ton lorries grinding by, while I watched from across the road.

The aim was to engage him – he agreed to let them fetch some shopping for him and, crucially, to meet them again the next week – win his trust and work towards providing him with the treatment he needs in the community.

But when I described this scenario to a London psychiatrist, he responded 'They (the professionals) must be mad. They will find themselves in front of an enquiry panel when that man injures someone'. Thus does fear drive the system, inhibiting innovation and encouraging incarceration as the 'safe' option?

One consequence has been growing protest from the people who use the services. The rise of the consumer's movement in mental health is the most striking development of the last ten years.

Laurance, Mental Health: The Fear Factory,
The Independent on Sunday, 30th June 2002: p18.

The issue of dangerous people with severe personality disorders complicates an issue which is already controversial enough. *The Independent on Sunday*'s editorial (30th June 2002: p22) opines that: 'this Bill threatens to turn mental hospitals into prisons to reassure the public that it is safe from largely imaginary perils'. Of course, the murder of Lynne and Megan Russell, and the murder of Sophie Hook in Llandudno were by people who were clearly mentally disordered, albeit in a form which is not easy to define, and were seen as almost inevitably going to be a risk to the limb and life of others by those who had come into contact with them. Any government cannot simply ignore the threat which in the case of Sophie Hook led to local agencies saying in effect: 'we knew that he was going to do something dangerous but we have no powers to offer him help and protect the innocent.'

Shaun Russell, husband of Lin and father of Megan and Jose, is quoted in *The Times* in a statement which sums up many of the dilemmas facing government, professionals and the public:

These measures (on DSPD) are good in the sense that perhaps if they had been in place at the time when Michael Stone attacked my family it might have meant that it did not happen.

But I would be very keen to see that the measures were trialled and tested so that there is a minimal chance of people being wrongfully detained. There is a civil liberties issue to consider. But I cannot get it out of my mind that if these measures had been in place, it might have saved my family.

The Times, 26th June 2002: p10.

A factor which has not come into the media debate, but is something about which professionals, especially social workers, are very aware, is the fact that many people with a mental illness as defined by the 1983 Act, but with other complicating factors of substance misuse, difficult personality etc., were often denied the treatment that they needed and often wanted. Some psychiatrists were in the habit of changing people's labels, e.g. from schizophrenia to personality disorder, so that the 'treatability' clause in the 1983 Act meant that they no longer had clinical responsibility for them. As Health Minister, Jacqui Smith, stated recently:

> This means that people with personality disorders will no longer be **excluded** from compulsory treatment on the grounds that they are untreatable, provided they meet the criteria for compulsion.
> quoted in *Community Care*, 27th June, 2002: p6 (my emphasis).

The role and value of the Approved Social Worker (ASW)

> The message that comes through from these visits (by the Mental Health Act Commission) is that the role of the ASW in the care of patients with acute mental illness is crucial. Almost without exception, case notes, interviews, and discussions with users and carers demonstrate that the early and continuing involvement of a skilled and committed ASW can make all the difference between a patient being caught up in a revolving door of short periods in the community interspersed with enforced stays in acute units, or being able to lead a less restricted life with only a rare need for in-house patient care.
> Margaret Clayton, chairperson, Mental Health Act Commission, *Community Care*, 23rd May, 2002: p38.

> Approved social workers should have a wider role than reacting to requests for admission to hospital, making the necessary arrangements and ensuring compliance with the law.
> DHS Circular no. LAC (86) 15, para. 14.

Already it will be plain from our historical survey that one of the main values that the ASW brings to this complex process of assessment is their independence:

- Their operation as independent professionals accountable for their own professional judgement.
- The fact that they are employed by an agency which is **not** part of the NHS.
- The fact that their employing authority has responsibilities and connections with a wide variety of social and educational agencies.

Added to the above, are a number of other valuable aspects:

- Holistic skills in a whole person/whole systems assessment.
- A social and environmental perspective.
- Post-qualifying experience.
- Specific training.
- Ability in working in partnership with individuals, families and agencies.

> It's not just about doing the ASW training, its social work training and perspectives from the beginning.
> approved social worker.

The British Association of Social Workers suggested in its evidence in the lead up to the 1983 Act that the role of the ASW in compulsory admissions should be:

- To investigate the client's social situation and how that has developed; and to estimate, in consultation with others involved, the extent to which the social and environmental pressures have contributed to the client's observed behaviour.
- To apply professional skill to help modify any contributory personal relationship or environmental factors.
- To mobilise the resources of the health services, the community service, and acknowledge and use the community as a therapeutic resource.
- To ensure that any intervention is the least restrictive necessary in the circumstances.
- To ensure strict compliance with the law.
  BASW, Review of the Mental Health Act, 1959, *Further Evidence*, 1980: p25.

This role is currently being undertaken not only within the context of a debate around the reform of the legislation, but increasing policy guidance and research. The recent guidance on *Adult Acute In-patient Care Provision*, (April 2002), quotes the MIND enquiry as stating that:

> In-patient services must be conceived as stepping-stones to inclusion, not departure points for exclusion. The ultimate aim is participation in the mainstream of society for all who desire it.
> *Creating Accepting Communities*, Report of the MIND Enquiry, 1998–99.

This is a vital precept regarding the social work role, as the ASW is in an extremely influential position to see the individual within their whole person, familial, community, social contexts; assess their needs; look for the least restrictive environment for care; and follow through with

Table 7: Social work and ASW roles and their overlap.

Social Work Role	Social Work and ASW Role	ASW Role
Generic role	Assessment skills	Technical, specialist knowledge
Social perspective	Interviewing skills	Legal/social orientation
Shared responsibility	Providing support	Semi-autonomous
Broad remit	Interaction across boundaries of legislation and services e.g. mental health, childcare, disability, old age etc.	Narrow remit
Planning toward future or aftercare		Concentration on current crisis, but need to link before and after
Team worker	Acting in interests of user	independent practitioner

Derived from Ulas and Connor, 2000: p96.

the individual. The recent Sainsbury Centre executive briefing on Adult In-patient Care (Briefing 16, June 2002) stresses the need to combat the 'disconnection from the system of care as a whole' which so often happens for people on admission, and makes a number of pertinent comments around attitudes, approaches, staff development and leadership. The Sainsbury Centre for Mental Health, in partnership with the Department of Health, the Royal College of Psychiatrists, the Royal College of Nursing and the NHS Confederation has begun a new project – *The Search for Acute Solutions*; and the recent Mental Health Foundation Survey of alternatives to acute hospital in-patient admission is also helpful here (*Being There In A Crisis*, February, 2002).

> *While the extension of the psychosocial approach has increased health professionals' awareness of social care issues, social workers bring a unique perspective that can counter-balance the rather individualistic focus of their health colleagues.*
> director of mental health services, clinical psychology background.

Marion Ulas and Anne Connor in their work on the Scottish system set out a very useful model of the social work role, the Mental Health Officer (Scotland's version of the ASW) role and the overlap between them:

To fulfil these complex roles well and to safeguard the interests of the individual while at the same time ensuring proper attention to risk and safety, requires enormous skill and indeed courage. At the first National Institute for Mental Health in England conference at the end of June 2002, there was an interesting workshop on the reform of the Mental Health Act. Listening in to the groups within the workshop and taking soundings wider within the conference, it became clear that ASWs' anxieties

over the possible loss of their role was echoed in concerns from other professionals about taking it over. Nurses and nurse managers emphasised their focus on the individual, one-to-one therapeutic relationship with their service users. One nurse manager was crystal clear in his view that while nurses could fulfil the Approved Mental Health Professional role as envisaged in the reform proposals; he felt that they would be very reluctant to carry it out. 'Let's face it', he said to me, 'social workers have a record of standing up to medics, and there are many times when they have stopped compulsory admission and found a proper and appropriate alternative. Nurses fear that the use of statutory powers will blight their therapeutic relationship with their users', (nurse manager to author, June 2002). One experienced ASW within the workshop on mental health legislation said that her experience with working with respected community nurse colleagues had changed her mind. She now felt that nurses would be able to take on that role. Interestingly, however, one of the nurses in the group stated clearly that:

'(The use of statutory powers) could jeopardise my relationship with the patient'. Another ASW made the point which is extremely relevant and recognisable to social workers, especially those in the Mental Health and Childcare fields. 'Social workers', he said, 'have had to cope with the turbulence within the therapeutic relationship of using statutory powers'. Indeed, the evidence from Mental Health and Childcare is that if statutory powers are used courteously, sensitively and effectively, the relationship is usually not harmed, and can indeed be enhanced. This is not, however, an easy concept to take on board.

> *I never yet met a nurse who wished to exercise statutory powers.*
> mental health trainer.

Section13 (2) of the 1983 Act lays a duty on the ASW to interview the user 'in a suitable manner' and it is the awareness of personal, familial, social and cultural factors, and the person-to-person listening skills, described in Chapter 5, which come into play here.

Margaret Clayton, Chairperson of the Mental Health Act Commission in a recent article in *Community Care* draws attention to the key role the ASW has in the following tasks under the Act:

- Emergency admissions under Section 4 of the Act.
- The outcome of detention under Section 136 of the Act.
- The granting of authorised leave under Section 17.
- Arrangements for aftercare under Section 117.

In the 9th Biennial report, 1999-2001, by the Commission, the point is made that:

> *The role is also widely seen as providing a safeguard against unnecessary admission by bringing in a balancing, non-medical view of the best interests of the patient and the need to use the least restricted alternative available to provide care.*
> Mental Health Act Commission, 2001: para. 2.47).

The Commission goes on to say that:

> *The ASW's role is therefore complex and, at times, beset with problems of both practice and principle. However, we continue to believe that ASWs play a vital role in the administration of the Act. If an equivalent role in new legislation is to be undertaken by a wider professional group (such as community-based nurses), we urge the government to consider how the benefits of the current structure might be protected.*
> para. 2.48.

The 'crucial role' (Clayton, *Community Care*, p39) of 'ensuring that patients are not granted authorised leave unless robust arrangements are in place for their care outside the acute unit', is also highlighted by Clayton, and a distressing number of suicides occur while the patient is on authorised leave. This was, of course, also an issue in the Benjamin Rathbone enquiry, already referred to in this book, in which the social worker was the professional most persistent in highlighting the dangers.

It would seem right to give the last word in this section to an ASW. In an e-mail of May 2002, this experienced practitioner made the following points:

- Social workers in Mental Health operate on the margins.

- One of the main themes throughout the training of the ASW is their status as an independent practitioner, independent not only from the doctors who may be involved in an assessment, but also from any overriding sense of obligation to their own employer. The ASW is freed up to act in the best interests of the service user and to apply the guidance contained within the Act and the Code of Practice.
- This unusual level of autonomy is pivotal to the role, which was intended to provide a fail safe against inappropriate use of the powers of detention. A counterbalance to the draconian powers which can allow the removal of liberty without the scrutiny of the courts.
- I would argue that by and large the ASWs have been effective in providing an informed and 'critically supportive' role in the assessment of people with mental health needs. The relationship with doctors is predominantly one of mutual respect and acceptance, there may be differences of opinion, but they are usually in the context of debate rather than conflict.
- Often in such circumstances, the ASW is left with two medical recommendations and total responsibility for any course of action other than detention in hospital – it can be a lonely role.

> *The ASW is there to give a broader view than a purely medical model. Mental health is not something that can be looked at in purely clinical terms.*
> Hywel Williams, MP, one of the UK's first ASWs, Quoted in *Community Care*, 4th July 2002, p19.

The strength that the ASW brings to the assessment process is a knowledge of the circumstances, the networks and the resources, which is usually significantly more comprehensive than that provided by the medical input. The knowledge of the ASW can be a significant factor in the successful use of alternatives to hospital admission.

The ASW is tasked with a co-ordination and management function – they are in charge of the process of assessment. The 'stage management' of the assessment is a skilled and time-consuming task that has a major impact on both the outcome, the level of risk, and the service user's perspective of the process.

The management of the process involves the co-ordination of a range of agencies and informal participants, often in the setting of crisis and florid behaviour.

The task is often to hold a difficult and sometimes dangerous situation and to maintain control with little in the way of resources in settings which may not be suited to the purpose. It is a skilled job.

In fulfilling this task, the ASW will be called to draw upon the whole range of interpersonal skills. They may be required to use an awareness of group dynamics (assessments are often in the setting of dynamic group settings). They will be expected to maintain an anti-discriminatory approach. They will need to use their interviewing skills. Most of all, they will need to develop an accurate assessment of all the circumstances surrounding the crisis and to form a clear view upon which to take a decision. They must then relay their decision to the service user directly.

> *ASWs are the only people in the mental health process to take an holistic approach and actively protect the rights of the individual. They are able to do so because they are independent – they are not accountable to hospitals or social services departments, only to the law.*
>
> Paul Jewitt, ASW, quoted in *Community Care*, 4th July 2002: p19.

- 'Sectioning' people are the tip of the iceberg. The ASW is also a key player in the CPA process and should have a lead role in the care planning and the after care implementation for the service user, whether they are detained or not. The ASW has been a prime mover in the development of community services for people with mental health needs, which have reduced social isolation and have provided a sense of purpose and structure in the lives of some people who otherwise would have little to brighten their existence.
- Over the years, a number of components which characterised the work of ASWs have been assumed by other professions or groups. This has had a wider gain for people using mental health services, with the growth of counselling, befriending etc. services, but the therapeutic side of the ASW role has tended to get lost, leaving the statutory core behind.
- The statutory work of the ASW has appeared less attractive to takeover bids. There has been a widespread reluctance to take on this role, both from individuals and also from Health as an organisation. Health has significant difficulties in adopting the social control

elements of mental health work. They are philosophically out of tune with the use of statute as a mechanism for ensuring that individuals who have lost their own sense of personal control are offered care and control.

- The local authority is an organisation much more experienced and accustomed to the use of statutory powers to oblige the unwilling to conform to societal expectations and obligations. In some respects, the ASW has much more in common with colleagues in child protection than they may have with their Health Service counterparts. The link with the local authority is an important safeguard to the ASW, who although acting as an independent professional, may need the backing and support of an organisation which is at ease with defending decisions where compulsion through statute has been a feature.
- Any reform of the Mental Health Act will need an ASW-type role. Someone needs to co-ordinate the process of assessment, and in instances of compulsory admission there is a vital role in 'owning' the process and seeing it through to a conclusion. The ASW is the only person who maintains involvement from the point of referral (or earlier) to the conclusion of admission. Their role in the tribunal scrutiny of detention is also vital.

There are issues of maintaining independence, and the role issues and culture around the interaction between doctors and nurses is an issue for the introduction for the new approved mental health professional. In a world where the issue of treatability has become so prevalent, there is still a vital role for the 'reasonable person' role in mental health assessment. This is both as a guardian to liberty for people who are behaving strangely but are not mentally ill (see the case examples around Section 136) and also to ensure that people who are mentally disordered and dangerous, but do not fit into a neat clinical category, are offered the care and control that they and the public need. The ASW can help doctors to consider other perspectives and to form a view 'through the invaluable process of debate'. (I am indebted to Colin Farnworth, ASW and Manager with Staffordshire Social Services for his thoughts which led to the above section.)

It cannot be emphasised too strongly that the Mental Health Act Commission, the successor to the Earl of Shaftesbury's original commission to protect the rights of individuals with a mental illness in various forms of care and custody, have consistently praised the role of the ASW.

The recent newspaper debate around the proposed reform of the 1983 Act demonstrates that the debate around liberty and safety is nowhere near to reaching a state of equipoise. Demokritus, the Greek philosopher, stated that people would always choose a state of liberty over and above a state of comfortable and safe tyranny, but today's public, with rising expectations, tend to demand both! It was Alexis de Tocqueville in his *Democracy in America* (1835) who pointed out that the new tyranny in democracies could well be that of public opinion.

If the envisaged Approved Mental Health Professional is not effective, then the gate-keeping role is passed to the new tribunals, but, as compulsory detention will have already taken place, the gate moves from the point of detention to the point before treatment, and this is an issue which will almost immediately start a new debate from the inception of a new Act.

As the Sainsbury Centre in its Briefing 14 (March 2001) asserts on 'the role of social work':

> *A number of current policy proposals are putting the social work model in Mental Health Services under threat, and there is a danger that this perspective could be lost by default unless this is addressed. Loss of the social work model from the process of detention would be a major step backwards. There is a danger that the understandable decision not to retain the role of the Approved Social Worker will lead to a narrowing of the focus when the evidence and the other policy points to a more comprehensive approach to assessing and addressing users' needs.*
>
> p8.

The future

Bearing in mind the shortage of approved social workers, and the changing nature of their deployment, it is understandable that the proposals for the reform of the Act have introduced the new Approved Mental Health Professional. Both the Association of Directors of Social Services (ADSS) and BASW have acknowledged that there are problems with the current system, and the BASW Mental Health Special Interest Group in its proposals dated the 28th May 2002, set out the difficulties facing ASWs at the present time:

- A 64 per cent increase in the number of assessments over the last ten years set against a static or declining number of ASWs.

- Assessments are becoming more protracted and more stressful with an increasing level of violence, and a difficulty in obtaining second medical recommendations.
- The time now being spent on assessments makes it difficult for ASWs to carry out their casework role (see also the comments in the section above).
- In areas where there is a lack of crisis intervention services, ASWs are often at the pressure point and the 'first port of call' for carers and other agencies.
- In places where acute services are under-resourced, ASWs often find themselves trapped between the demands of carers or other agencies and the unavailability of a hospital bed.
- ASWs find themselves in an increasingly exposed position legally.
- Their incorporation into joint provider services, in the new Trusts, has compromised their legal and professional independence.

Many social workers say that they receive good supervision and support within the new management arrangements, but ASWs are the least satisfied by the new arrangements, feeling that their specific needs have *not* been addressed.

As we have seen from the historical sweep of issues around liberty and safety, the whole thrust of English law is to provide checks and balances to legal processes. The questions that must be answered around the changing nature of this 'balancing' role will be:

- Is there sufficient independence?
- Is there an holistic perspective?
- Are there people available to undertake the role?

Currently, most ASWs are seconded to mental health trusts but are retained in employment by their local authority. This will be difficult to maintain over time and also it will be increasingly difficult to assert their independence within the legal framework.

I share the BASW approach that there needs to be a new animal. BASW proposes someone called a Mental Health Act Officer (MHAO) who would take over the quasi-legal element of the present ASW role.

The MHAO might come from a number of professions, but must have had the same level of experience as the current ASWs, and must also undergo the same type and amount of training.

The holistic and social perspectives in the assessment process **must** be retained and enhanced.

The MHAO would have to be employed in their role as a statutory agent by a public body which would **not** be a provider of mental health services. BASW proposes that it could be a consortium of NHS and Local Authority commissioners, overseen by the new Commission for Mental Health. Variations on a theme could be a body similar to CAFCASS, who have taken on board the duties of the Guardians ad Litem from local authorities.

Whatever the constitution of the body, it must be demonstrably **separate** and **independent** of mental health providers, who are increasingly large organisations covering populations of about a million people. If the issues of independence and skills are not handled adroitly in the current climate, then the pendulum between liberty and safety which is oscillating at an alarming speed at present will continue. One only needs to look at the press coverage of cause célèbres in the period between the 1845 Act and that of 1890 (see Jones K, 1972: Chapters 6 and 7), and consider the much more prevalent power of the media today, to see how this vital role needs to be appropriately translated into the new legislation.

In the autumn of 2002 I took part in a number of seminars concerning the Mental Health Bill. It was illuminating just how supportive of the ASW role, and the social worker's values and skills within that role, were other professionals: psychiatrists (including notably the President of the Royal College of Psychiatrists, Dr Mike Shooter), specialist lawyers, nurses (especially those involved in monitoring Mental Health Act admissions). The checks and balances in the system are an essential component in British governance, and in mental health law it is the ASW who provides one of those vital checks on executive power. At the Eastern Regional Conference on the Mental Health Bill (see Eastern Development Centre of NIMHE, *The Draft Mental Health Bill – Radical Enough?* 11th September 2002) Professor Peter Jones, Practising Psychiatrist and academic from Cambridge University, described the ASW as 'the essential grit in the oyster, helping to produce the pearl of positive outcomes for users'. We must retain the 'grit' to continue producing 'pearls'.

Chapter 7

The Value of Social Work in Management and Leadership

The modernisation of mental health services is a complex and demanding task. It requires strong leadership and clarity of vision which encompasses both long and short-term goals. It also requires effective and inclusive management and planning structures.
Social Services Inspectorate Report. *Modernising Mental Health Services*, June 2002: para 6.1.

Trust and credibility comes through everyone's observation of the manager's symbolic integrity, not his or her 'policy document'.
Tom Peters, 1987: p149.

What makes a significant difference to the performance of an organisation is the quality and competence of front-line managers.
Denise Platt, Chief Inspector of the SSI, Annual Report, 1999.

The role of the corporate leader is to manage conflicting needs in a synergistic way, creating an environment in which opposing forces can be reconciled to create rapid and strong growth.
Charles Hampden-Turner, 1990: p11.

Leadership is about working through others to achieve a vision.
Penny Humphries, Acting Director, NHS Leadership Centre.

In this life you have to be your own hero. By that I mean you have to win whatever it is that matters to you by your own strength and in your own way.
Jeanette Winterson, 2000: p155.

Excitable, anxious, extreme, obstinate, jealous or oversuspicious, he [sic] must not be. Such a man [sic] is never at rest. The leader must so arrange everything

that the strong have something to yearn for and the weak nothing to run from.
Benedict of Nursia, Chapter 64.

Senior managers of today's large enterprises must move beyond strategy, structure and systems to a framework built on purpose, process and people.
Bartlett and Ghoshal, 1994: p79.

Two sides of the same coin

Having been a practitioner, a frontline manager and a senior manager in organisations, I find it both sad and infuriating when practitioners and managers engage in postures of mutual incomprehension. As Terry Scragg and I made clear in our publication *Managing to Care*, practice and management are two sides of the same coin, (Gilbert and Scragg, 1992). Practitioners, especially those who work in organisations, delivering statutory and organisational requirements, and working to help their clients negotiate complicated routes through society's systems, have to be good at managing themselves, managing the therapeutic relationship (and I don't mean controlling it!), and managing the environment. Social workers in the mental health field have to manage their own personal system; work/life balance, emotions, the balance between the emotional, the cognitive, the creative, the spiritual and the physical; they need to be able to manage their time and to interact in an effective way across a range of partnerships. Their management of the therapeutic relationship is not one of control but of clarity in agreeing shared outcomes, and enabling a vulnerable and perhaps chaotic individual to stick to those agreed objectives. As Gerard Egan has written: 'Helpers are seen as competent because they are active, because they listen intently . . . talk intelligently . . . are understanding, genuine and respectful'. In all this, Egan argues that: 'helpers must be able to **deliver**'. (Egan, 1986, quoted in Gilbert and Scragg, 1992: p112 (my emphasis).)

The Greek Xenophon (writing in the 4th century BC) believed that there was small risk of a leader being 'regarded with contempt . . . if whatever he may have to preach, he shows himself best able to perform'. In this respect, leadership in the multi-disciplinary setting is

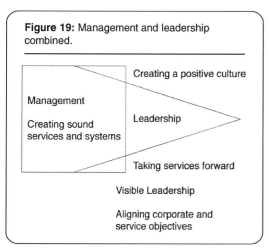

Figure 19: Management and leadership combined.

Management
Creating sound services and systems

Creating a positive culture

Leadership

Taking services forward

Visible Leadership

Aligning corporate and service objectives

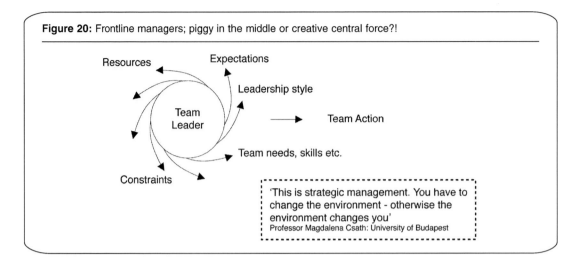

Figure 20: Frontline managers; piggy in the middle or creative central force?!

Resources   Expectations

Leadership style

Team Leader   ⟶   Team Action

Team needs, skills etc.

Constraints

'This is strategic management. You have to change the environment - otherwise the environment changes you'
Professor Magdalena Csath: University of Budapest

complex, as managers with training in one discipline will be leading staff from other disciplines. Managers do not have to be the most proficient practitioner, but they have to have and demonstrate empathy with the end users (whether we're talking care service or business), with their frontline staff and managers and backup staff. The larger and more complex the organisation, the wider the range of professional experts there will be who have to be nurtured and directed to work towards the goals of the organisation. Flamholtz and Randle (1989) set out three key requirements for playing the inner game of management successfully (see also Gilbert and Thompson, 2002):

1. Being able to manage your own self-esteem so that you derive satisfaction from the things managers are supposed to do, that is enabling rather than doing.
2. Being able to manage your need for direct control over people and results.
3. Being able to manage your need to be liked so that it does not interfere with performing the managerial role.

Chris Payne, in a short article, which still is an excellent read for frontline managers, comments that:

It is a sad fact that there are many residential managers who interpret their role either in terms of 'doing' all the things for which their staff are paid to do or who become administrators pure and simple. Instead of which they should be building on their knowledge and understanding of practice to take a more rounded and prospective view of the services being offered; to initiate sensitive programmes of, for example, staff recruitment and selection, development, supervision, training and

stress management; to create a sound 'foreign policy' for their establishment; and most importantly to offer skilled professional leadership to staff.

Payne, 1988.

If practitioners sense that their manager is not a leader in the real sense of path-finding with individuals and groups towards common goals (see Gilbert and Thompson, 2002), but rather has their eye purely on the bottom line, especially if it's the bottom line of his or her own ambition(!), then they will be disinclined to see them as real leaders and to follow them.

One of the major interactions between practice and management is at the frontline manager level; in this instance the management of community mental health teams, day opportunity services, supported living services etc. Forging genuine two-sided coins of practice and management is an essential function of senior management. Frontline managers are in a potentially very creative, but also possibly very invidious position, and must be helped to blend the best of practice and management together.

When one looks at the conclusions from the findings of research into the integration of health and social services in Somerset (Gulliver, Peck and Towell, June 2002) it is very evident that it is vital to ensure that leadership is seen as a concept for all staff and for all partners in the enterprise. Especially if one looks at the management of risk that practitioners and managers have to engage in, leadership is an essential component here.

Case example 9 demonstrates just how much leadership is involved in enabling people with potential to harm themselves or others to lead as independent a life as possible. A former Director of Social Services and Chief Executive of a major voluntary organisation perceived the dichotomy between practitioner and manager as one that is often artificially constructed:

Social workers have to take very tough decisions . . . All of this is a strong school for decision-making. Social worker skills are eminently transferable to a management environment.

quoted in Fielding, 1989.

Managers in mental health services need to be aware of the major environmental factors affecting the work that they are undertaking, without becoming overwhelmed by those same factors. The STEP process, enables one to chart the major influencing factors (see Gilbert and Thompson, 2002, for more detail):

- Sociological
  - increased consumer power
  - demographic changes
  - multiculturalism and culture/creed tensions
  - marginalisation of some groups
- Technological
  - faster (but not always better) communication
  - technological innovation
  - cross-fertilization of ideas
  - need for quicker responses across a range of areas
- Economic
  - a knowledge-based economy
  - market uncertainty, post Enron and Worldcom
  - increasing role of private sector finance
- Political
  - new political alliances post 11th September 2001
  - dangers of polarisation

All of this takes place in a globalised market place with increased opportunities and increased threats.

Change and faster change appears to be endemic, and there is a widespread belief that structural change will produce better performance but as Mark C. Scott demonstrates in his study of business organisations, the major structural changes have produced increasingly small returns (Scott, 2000), and as he states:

The problem with knowledge for most businesses and their boards is that it is intangible . . . it is personalised. It tends to walk out of the building each night!

p6.

Roger Harrison in his study of organisational culture is clear that:

. . . the organisation is a living organism . . . and the more you ask it to change, the less energy it will have available for its daily work. It behoves us to intervene no more 'deeply' than is required to obtain the desired competencies.

Harrison, 1990.

This is a message also reinforced by Edward Peck from the Institute for Applied Health and Social Policy, in his commentary in MCC (10: 3, June 2002) on the previous issue's study of case studies in integrated health and social care, namely that the lesson both from the private and the public sector is that mergers and acquisitions do not always bring tangible benefits for users and carers.

Organisational culture

Over the past century, there have been different ways of considering organisations and how one need to run them.

Zohar and Marshall propose five generations of business models:

1. the organisations as machines
2. organisations as systems
3. organisations as organisms (living systems)
4. organisations as emotional/social systems
5. organisations as fully human systems

Zohar and Marshall, 2000.

Most businesses and health and social care agencies have left the first evolutionary model – the organisation as machines – behind, but the culture within organisations varies markedly and has a profound effect on how organisations deliver services to the people they serve. Organisational culture is sometimes described as: 'the way we do things here', and in those simple terms one can often touch the culture within a team, ward, house, day service – or even within an organisation as a whole. Edgar Schein, the doyen of studies in organisational culture defines it as:

A pattern of basic assumptions – invented, discovered, or developed by a given group as it learned to cope with its problems of external adaptation and internal integration – that is worked well enough to be considered valid and, therefore, to be taught to new members as the correct way to perceive, think and feel in relation to those problems.

Schein, 1985: p9.

For a fuller discussion of the subject, please see Gilbert and Thompson, 2002: pages 2.85–2.91.

Case Example 12

Dangerous liaison

Declan Henry faced a tough task in trying to rehabilitate a murderer and habitual drug user. His client, who stabbed his father to death, refuses to acknowledge that he has a mental illness, and is expressing a hatred of his mother.

Case notes
The name of the client has been changed.
Practitioner: Declan Henry
Field: Deputy manager of a forensic rehabilitation unit for mentally disordered offenders
Location: London
Client: George Kemp, aged 36.
Case history: Kemp has been diagnosed with paranoid schizophrenia and has a paranoid personality disorder. He also has a long-standing habitual drug problem. In 1988, he murdered his father, stabbing him 26 times. He said he felt emotionally abused by his father, who had become an 'object of hate' in his life. On being discharged from hospital, Kemp lived for two-and-a-half years in the community. But in 1997 he was recalled to hospital after his mother reported him for growing marijuana in his back garden, since when he has been detained in a medium secure unit (under section 37/41 of the Mental Health Act 1983). Efforts to implement his deferred conditional discharge have failed since November 1999 owing to his refusal to follow his care plan and his continued drug misuse.
Dilemma: Kemp's unrealistic expectations and, at times, limited view of reality may well set him up to fail, but – given his institutionalisation – may also be deliberately contrived precisely to fail.
Risk factor: Kemp's inability to accept his mental illnesses, drug misuse, and his growing hatred towards his mother may put himself and others at risk of serious harm.
Outcome: Kemp's overnight stays at the rehabilitation unit have been successfully completed without attempts to sabotage the care plan and with signs of drug use.

When Declan Henry became the keyworker to George Kemp, a murderer with diagnosed paranoid schizophrenia and a paranoid personality disorder, and attendant drug habit, he knew he had his hands full.

Not just because of the challenge presented by Kemp's case, but also because he was a murderer – or rather, because of his murder victim. Henry, deputy manager of a voluntary-run forensic rehabilitation unit, had recently suffered the trauma of his own father's death through natural causes, and here was a client who, in 1988, had brutally murdered his father by stabbing him 26 times: 'The loss I was feeling for my own father clashed with the sometimes cavalier attitude that he had towards killing his father,' Henry recalls.

His own feelings aside, Henry identified three main risks with Kemp: his habitual drug-taking, his violent history, and his lack of understanding of his mental illness.

'Since being accepted in September 2001, he has sabotaged his placement by taking crack cocaine on at least three occasions,' says Henry. 'And if he was able to get hold of crack cocaine in a medium secure hospital, out here the opportunity is considerably greater. It's not a restricted unit. Clients have their own front-door key. Kemp will have to reside here at night in line with Home Office restrictions, but can come and go as he pleases.'

Kemp finally began his 'afternoon leave' in January. Again, the omens were not good. 'On his return from his first unescorted visit,' recalls Henry, 'he tested positive for cannabis and possibly another substance. We gave him a final warning – any more and the offer of a placement would be withdrawn.'

Henry considers that his sabotage tactic may be deliberate: 'Maybe there is a lot of anxiety about coming out of an institution,' he says. But this is where the unit usually comes into its own. 'We work with very difficult clients and we have a heavy emphasis on life skills, which we teach them so they can move on to less supported accommodation or an independent flat,' says Henry. 'Ideally, they stay with us for between 18 months and two years. We don't usually look at clients moving on until they have been here at least a year.'

Kemp's perception of reality was, not surprisingly, blurred. He had monthly depot injections (see Factfile, page 41) but complained that they caused trembling as a side-effect. 'He doesn't feel he has a mental health problem and wants to stop having the injections,' says Henry. 'He feels he was mentally ill at the time of his father's murder, but that his psychotic illness was induced by drugs. He says he is remorseful about the offence but does not feel responsible because he was unwell at the time. At other times he is not remorseful.'

The forensic psychiatrist recommended Kemp's medication remain unaltered given the major change about to happen in his life. 'We felt a review would be more appropriate later on depending on his progress,' says Henry.

Kemp's violent history was also a crucial factor. He had been violent towards fellow patients but not staff. He hadn't spoken to his mother after she informed on him, since when she has replaced his father as his new object of hate. She is 'in hiding' in France.

Kemp – who has attempted suicide twice and has self-harmed at least three times over the past 10 years – was very capable of hostility. 'My first experience came when I attempted to address his drug problem,' says Henry, who admits his forthright tactics were possibly stirred by memories of his own father. Kemp's initial response was: 'I no longer have a drug problem – it's in the past.' But Henry knew he had taken drugs six weeks previously, and had spent over £28,000 on crack cocaine (he rented out a flat he owned) and was in debt with a bank loan. 'In retrospect,' says Henry, I feel I went too far,' he concedes, 'and our relationship deteriorated. He was angry with me for challenging him and I felt inadequate as a practitioner by his response to my approach.'

At a three-way clear-the-air meeting Henry, his manager and Kemp discussed these difficulties, with Kemp eventually accepting that Henry would remain as his keyworker.

The relationship has clearly improved. Kemp, aware of the expectations placed upon him, has begun his twice-weekly overnight stays and has remained drug-free. Henry is confident that Kemp's full-time trial period will soon begin. 'Our main source of work from now on will be containment. It doesn't sound like much, but given the complexity of a client like this, it will be an achievement,' says Henry.

Arguments for risk

- Kemp has displayed an ability to live in the community in relative safety, but was unable to deal effectively with his drug use. Targeted work within this area could lead to a successful transition.
- He has, at times, shown remorse for killing his father and has blamed his mental illness for his actions.
- Kemp has been institutionalised for a long time and the thought of having to deal with the outside world may be at the root of his attempts to sabotage his community placement. Skilled help could see him overcome this fear.
- Kemp is stable and well. Henry is confident that he is capable of making a focused effort to deal with his situation positively.
- Living in an environment that permits freedom of movement (excepting the need to remain at the unit at night) allows Kemp some independence and choice that would be denied him in hospital.

Arguments against risk

- Kemp is a murderer and habitual drug user. He has at times displayed a less-than-remorseful attitude to the murder. He has also, time and time again, relapsed into drug use from cannabis

(which is potentially harmful considering his mental health and medication) to crack cocaine.
- He can seemingly obtain drugs relatively easily – even when a patient at a medium-secure hospital. Moving him into a more independent lifestyle will only raise the temptation and access to drugs.
- Kemp is very able to scheme and manipulate. Challenged by Henry, he demanded that he be removed as his keyworker. This could indicate an unwillingness to tackle his behaviour constructively.
- If living more independently, there is a real risk that Kemp will stop his depot injections.
- As the new object of hate in his life, his mother is clearly at risk from harm. Although she is in hiding, she may return or, indeed, Kemp may try to find her.

Independent comment

Henry's approach demonstrates the value and centrality of a therapeutic relationship, writes Tom Dodd. It is understandable that the weight of Kemp's history alone (it has been 14 years since he killed his father) would tip the balance in favour of a containing and less-flexible regime.

The experience of paranoid disorders often means that the individual is less likely to take responsibility or see their role in the detrimental things that happen in their lives. Kemp may find it difficult to get pleasure from relationships, he may construe any comments as criticisms and blame the 'persecutor'. As his keyworker, Henry will need to take a cautious but intensive approach, while at a pace that is acceptable to Kemp because he is likely to disengage easily. If the aim of intervention is to modify Kemp's beliefs and behaviour, then he is less likely to fail.

The service's relationship with Kemp is likely to be over a period of years. To maintain opportunities for Kemp, the keyworker will need continued and comprehensive support from the multidisciplinary team. The care package is complex and will need a detailed rationale, with contributions from a number of sources. Such decision-making requires transparency and clarity from everyone involved. The more risks that are evident – and this case highlights many – the greater the imperative to take a team approach, sharing decision-making, accountability and responsibility.

Tom Dodd is co-ordinator for assertive outreach at the Sainsbury Centre for Mental Health.

Reprinted by kind permission of *Community Care*, 11–17 July, 2002.

In her study of culture in the public sector, Newman states that culture is learned and passed on from individual to individual or group:

> Culture is like language: we inherit it, learn it, pass it on to others, but in the process we invent new words and expressions – it evolves over time.
>
> Newman, 1996: p17.

Charles Handy famously described four cultures and labelled them with the names of Ancient Greek gods (see Handy, 1979 and 1985, 3rd edn. and Harrison and Stokes, 1990):

1. The power culture – frequently found in small entrepreneurial organisations. The system depends on a central power source (one person or a small coterie), 'with rays of power and influence spreading out from that central figure', (Handy, 1985: p189).
2. The role culture – central and local government departments fit the description for Handy's role culture. Its strengths are its stability and predictability, but at a time of change, that is its weakness as well.
3. The task culture – job or project orientated. Accent is on performance with a bringing together of the right people from any level in the organisation, with appropriate resources and setting them to get on with the task in hand.
4. The person culture – in this the individual is the central point. The structure exists only to serve and assist the individuals within it. Consultancies, barristers' chambers and architects' partnerships, are the type of organisations which Handy quotes as appropriate here.

Some general practitioner practices might well have fallen within the fourth culture, but in many ways, the formation of primary care groups and then primary care trusts were clearly created in part to bring GPs more into the organisational ring.

Cultures will change over time but they are notoriously slow to do so. Johnson and Scholes have a very helpful section on what they call the cultural web of an organisation based around a central 'recipe' and the ingredients comprising: rituals and myths, power structures, symbols, organisational structures, control systems and routines. To change the recipe in a large organisation is extremely difficult, though by changing some of the ingredients under the headings described will eventually lead to a modification, at least, of the recipe itself (see Johnson and Scholes, 1989, text and case studies, p37–47).

Edgar Schein makes clear that, in his opinion: 'the only thing of real importance that leaders do is to create and manage culture' (Schein, 1985: p2). If a newly arrived manager is aware of a service focused around organisational concerns rather than focused on positive outcomes for users and carers, or an organisation that is 'institutionally racist', then the leader's role is to change the recipe. Leaders, therefore, must:

- Identify the cultural recipe and how malleable it is.
- Diagnose its features and its layers.
- Ascertain how appropriate the recipe is for the desired strategy.
- Use transformational values and skills to mould the culture, by acting on the ingredients within the recipe. For example, managers going 'back to the floor' and working with frontline staff will not only inspire by example (walk-the-talk) and learn a great deal, they will also begin a weaving of stories and relationships which create a powerful force for positive development.

Management and leadership

Just as organisational theory was changing, so were the issues around management. Before the Second World War, there was a focus on 'administration' as an approach. This was characterised by mistake avoiding; rarely measuring performance; long hierarchies and limited delegation; risk avoiding; conformity and uniformity.

From the 1960s onwards, there was more of a focus on 'management', with objectives stated as broad strategic aim; performance measurement; shorter hierarchies and increased delegation; an active approach with a greater acceptance of risk and an accent on independence.

In the 1980s, 'leadership' theory was evolved to cope with an increasing environment of rapid change. Sir John Harvey-Jones makes a point which connects leadership and social work; in his words:

> Management and industrial leadership is an art, not a science. Each of us approaches the problem from a different background, and each of us is dealing with a different situation, and a different culture, and from a different starting point.
>
> Harvey-Jones, 1988: p27.

Table 8: The balancing foci of management and leadership.

The manager focuses on systems and structure	The leader focuses on people
The manager maintains	The leader develops
The manager asks how and when	The leader asks what and why
The manager concentrates on planning and budgeting	The leader sets a direction and aligns people
The manager has his eye on the bottom line	The leader has his eye on the horizon
The manager is deductive and rational	The leader is inductive and intuitive
The manager ensures the accomplishment of plans by controlling and problem solving	The leader achieves goals through motivating and inspiring people
Good management copes with current complexity	Leadership is about coping with change
The manager does things right	The leader does the right thing

Both facets are required for the organisation to flourish

Peter Gilbert, adapted from Kotter, What Leaders Really Do. *Harvard Business Review*, May/June 1990 and Bennis, Leadership in the 21st Century. *Journal of Organisational Change Management*, I: 1, 1989.

It might well be said that leadership is now being overstressed at the expense of management. Leadership is indeed required to take an organisation forward, but management is essential if the organisation is to work. Somebody once said that management and leadership are all about three interlocking activities: getting things right; keeping things going; doing new things! I tend to follow John P. Kotter who asserts that 'the real challenge is to combine strong leadership and strong management, and use each to balance the other'.

It is not always easy to combine the attributes of management and leadership in one person, though that may well be the ideal. If it's not possible then management teams need to be balanced to make sure that the correct skill mix is there.

> *What makes a significant difference to the performance of an organisation is the quality and competence of frontline managers. They manage the primary tasks and activities of the organisation. They have a key role in determining whether standards of practice are consistently maintained, in supporting staff engaged in complex, personally demanding practice, and ensuring that staff are continually developed in knowledge-based practice.*
> Denise Platt, Chief Inspector of the SSI,
> Annual Report 1999.

There are a number of theories of leadership:

- Leaders are born not made – charismatic leadership.
- Situational leadership which views leaders in the context of:
  - their own character and qualities
  - those of their subordinates
  - the situation at the time

- Theories based on the functions of leadership.

In this context, perhaps it is worth looking at what Penny Humphries, Acting Director of the NHS Leadership Centre believes leadership is about. 'Leadership', she said at a recent conference, 'is about working through others to achieve a vision'.

The characteristics of a leader could be viewed under three headings:

1. Personal: self-belief, self-awareness, a desire to drive improvement and integrity.
2. Setting direction: vision, intellectual flexibility, political astuteness and a drive for results.
3. Delivering improved services: leading change in an open and inclusive way, holding people to account and empowering others.
   Health Service Journal, 23rd May 2002: p14–5.

Jim Collins, in his recent study of enduringly successful organisations (and I stress enduring as opposed to the quick fix approach), points to leaders whose ambition is for the organisation and the service of their end users and not for themselves, (Collins, 2001). The recent collapse of Enron and Worldcom and the corporate scandals in America have led to many business thinkers and business schools to go back to fundamental issues such as values and consider what makes an organisation successful over a considerable time period. Jim Collins and Gerry Porras put it like this:

> *Contrary to popular wisdom, the proper first response to a changing world is not to ask, 'how should we change?' but rather to ask, 'what do we stand for and*

why do we exist?' This should never change. And then feel free to change everything else. Put another way, visionary companies distinguish their timeless core values and enduring purpose (which should never change) from their operating practices and business strategies (which should be changing constantly in response to a changing world).

Collins and Porras, 2000.

In this context, and the core categories which the Leadership Centre have set out, social work has a great deal to offer leadership both today and in the future in the following ways:

The leader looks out of the window to give praise and looks in the mirror to accept blame.

Jill Garrett, formerly European Director of Gallop.

1. Integrity and a sense of values

When interviewed for Community Care on her appointment as President of the ADSS, Jo Williams spoke of a 'fundamental' belief in equality, and treating everyone with the same respect as integral to her way of working both as a practitioner and as a senior manager. 'It's just part of me – how I am', is how she put it. (*Community Care*, 28th Oct. 1999) People who worked with Jo Williams as a social worker and a manager say that's exactly how she is. In management-speak she 'walks-the-talk'; unfortunately a number of people in senior positions are perceived as only being able to 'talk-the-talk'. They march to a different drum, that of their empty ambition.

It is not good enough just to preach the doctrine; you have to live the life.

Victoria Woodhull, US presidential candidate, 1872.

Stephen Covey in his work on principle-centred leadership argues for a congruency of personal, managerial and organisational principles:

Level	Principle
organisational	alignment
managerial	empowerment
interpersonal	trust
personal	trustworthiness

Covey, 1992.

As we have seen in Chapter 5, 'genuineness' is one of the prime attributes of the effective social worker. This is true for business leadership as well. Collins and Porras speak of 'core values' as the 'organisation's essential and enduring tenets – a small set of timeless guiding principles that require no external justification; they have *intrinsic* value and importance to those inside the organisation' (Collins and Porras, 2000, p222).

Collins, in his studies of leadership, is clear about a value-driven approach, concentrating on the good of the organisation, not the ambitions of the individual (Collins, 2001). Kouzes and Posner, in their overview of *The Credibility Factor: What Followers Expect From Their Leaders*, found that the responses to their survey of managers put integrity (trustworthiness) competence (capability and effectiveness) and leadership (direction-setting and inspiring) as the three most pronounced responses in that order (Kouzes and Posner, 1990.) Jack Welch, one of the most admired business leaders of his generation, recalls being asked how he could hold a particular belief system and be an effective businessman at the same time. Welch says that he answered emphatically that he could – 'the simple answer is', he stated, 'by maintaining integrity, establishing it and never wavering from it, supported everything I did through good and bad times. People may not have agreed with me on every issue, and I may not have been right all the time – but they always knew they were getting it straight and honest . . . I never had two agendas. There was only one way – the straight way' (Welch, with Byrne, 2001: p381. See also leadership case studies in Gilbert and Thompson, 2002.)

I have largely been very fortunate in the people I've worked for, but occasionally one comes up against somebody who can't even spell integrity let alone act with it. These are the 'hollow men', the 'Teflon' characters, who devalue the enterprises they and others are engaged in. They are not committed to the role and the organisation they are meant to be serving, but are intent on furthering their own career.

My favourite fictional/philosophical author, Ursula Le Guin, portrays such an individual in one of those children's books which have a lot to say to adults, *The Farthest Shore*. Cob, who had formerly been a mage engaged in doing good, had been corrupted by a desire to prolong his own life at the expense of others. His own rapacity for immortality was beginning to suck the life and colour out of the fabric of the universe. The mage who promotes life, Ged, challenges him in these words:

You exist, without name, without form. You cannot see the light of day; you cannot see the dark. You sold the green earth and the sun and the stars to save yourself. But you have no self. All that which you sold, that is yourself. You have given everything for nothing. And so now you seek to draw the world to you, all that life and life you lost, to fill up your nothingness. But it cannot be filled. Not all the songs of earth, not all the stars of heaven, could fill your emptiness.

Le Guin, 1973: p189.

At a time when business and business schools are having to re-evaluate their value-base in the light of the business and accountancy scandals in the United States, a profession which has a clear value-base and code of ethics, has a great deal to offer in today's world.

2. *Managing one's self*

As I said at the beginning of this chapter, practitioners, to be effective and helpful to others, have to manage themselves. They need to be self-aware, self-motivated, organised, dependable, and with a focus not only on positive outcomes for users and carers, but an awareness of their motivation for acting in a particular way.

As is the case in medicine, so it is for social work, the first injunction is to do no harm.

Think about the leaders you've been impressed with over the course of your working life. Almost without exception they will be people with high self-esteem, whose actions are congruent with their espoused views, who understand their own beliefs and values and who have a strong sense of their own direction. To be truly effective as a leader, you've got to be comfortable with who you are and what you are about. Essentially, concentrating on leading yourself is a powerful way to grow your ability to lead others.

Chris Lake, Programme Director, *Developing Leadership Potential*, Roffey Park Management Institute.

3. *Assessing situations*

One of the prime social work tasks is assessing the needs of individuals and care systems in a holistic manner. Social work assessments are not purely about an individual therapeutic relationship, as we have seen, they look at the individual in the context of their relationships and social circumstances.

Assessment of situations and possible consequences of actions or non-action is an essential part of leadership.

4. *Direction-setting*

When I joined the Army in the late 1960s, they had just engaged John Adair, to consider the interaction between historical and experiential views on leadership and the theoretical base. One of the simple models used by Adair and his successors and still very relevant today, is that of the famous three circles as set out below.

There is no doubt of the primacy of the mission or task; but of course it is usually

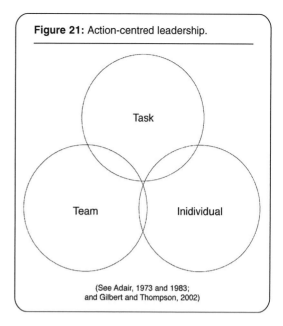

Figure 21: Action-centred leadership.

Task

Team   Inidividual

(See Adair, 1973 and 1983; and Gilbert and Thompson, 2002)

groups of people who are required to fulfil the mission, especially if it is complex and requires bringing in a number of specialists (Finance, IT, HR, etc.) whilst at the same time the team is only as strong as the weakest or least focused individual, and specialists may be brilliant in their own field but not particularly good 'team players'. The most effective social workers have to bring in to play, co-ordinate and influence a whole range of people from different professions and agencies. This is a good school of management. People with severe and enduring mental health needs, such as those surveyed in the Westminster Study (MacDonald and Sheldon, 1997) require a co-ordinated care package over a considerable period. Managing services which may be much dispersed and often out-sourced from the commissioning organisation, with staff out-posted and difficult to communicate with directly, require the manager to be extremely robust in making connections.

In Staffordshire, with a staff group of about 6,000 people, and with some of our most vital staff, home carers, for example, at the end of a long line of management and communication, we spent a considerable time when I was Director of Operations there, in ensuring a direct link between listening to our users and carers, managing strategically and involving those who were carrying out the day-to-day caring role.

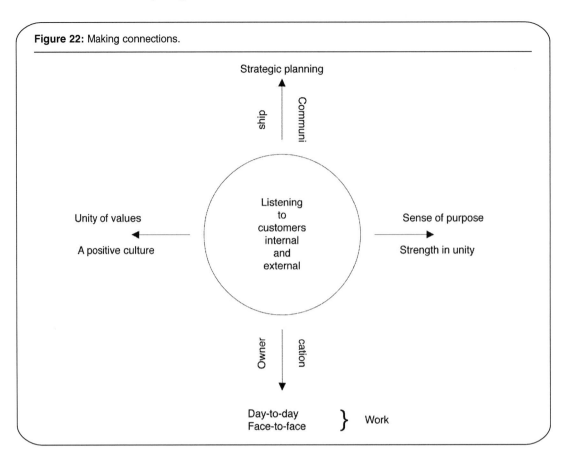

Figure 22: Making connections.

One of the main ways of ensuring performance is managed and evaluated, comes through the supervision process, which has been a common model for social work staff for many years, but is not so well known in other professional groups. Supervision integrates aims and tasks with the necessary development of attitude and aptitude within the staff member. Again, practice teaching, which is a well developed art in social work, and supervision, are good micro-management attributes.

5. *Creating a positive culture*

To operate successfully, social workers have to engage with people's cultural milieu – not only in terms of race and creed, but in the cultural web which we all weave within ourselves, around ourselves, within our immediate and extended families, and in the wider neighbourhood and society. The social worker has to understand what McLean and Marshall term 'a web of understanding', (McLean and Marshall, 1988: p11) and how various ingredients interact with the recipe as a

whole. Tom Peters is often quoted as saying that 'managing at any time, but more than ever today, is a symbolic activity', (see Peters and Austin, 1985, and Peters, 1989), while Smith and Peterson (1988) assert that the art of leadership resides significantly in the mediation of cultural messages between leaders and led.

In the complex organisational world of today, where public sector organisations are often vertically or horizontally linked with other public sector or private sector entities, the effectiveness of the leader lies in his/her ability to make activity meaningful for those around them.

Figure 24 moves action-centred leadership forward into today's world:

In an organisation which depends ultimately on interactions between people, then, as Charles Hampden-Turner points out in his book *Corporate Culture* (1990), leaders need to model behaviour for their staff. A number of service industries went to the public sector to gain ideas over caring for employees; now it may be that public sector organisations have to go back to learn from service industries. Well before Sven Goran Eriksson came into vogue, another

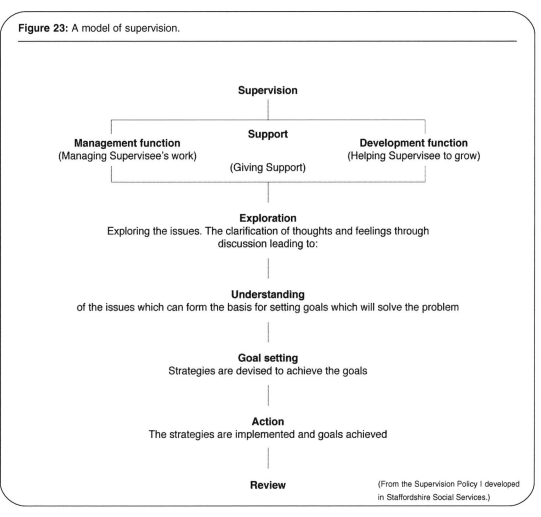

Figure 23: A model of supervision.

Supervision

Support

Management function
(Managing Supervisee's work)

(Giving Support)

Development function
(Helping Supervisee to grow)

Exploration
Exploring the issues. The clarification of thoughts and feelings through discussion leading to:

Understanding
of the issues which can form the basis for setting goals which will solve the problem

Goal setting
Strategies are devised to achieve the goals

Action
The strategies are implemented and goals achieved

Review

(From the Supervision Policy I developed in Staffordshire Social Services.)

Swede, Goran Carstedt, turned around Volvo France. His belief was that:

> You won't get your people to care about customers unless you show your people that you care about them. They'll pass on your concern. You don't 'motivate' your employees, you show them the concern you want them to express to customers.
>
> quoted in Hampden-Turner, 1990: p167.

6. Partnership and communication

It is a sad fact that sometimes positive and productive relations at the front line are sabotaged either by secrecy and/or conflict at a senior manager level between or within organisations, or at times good working relationships at a senior level which never get passed down to frontline staff through the middle management tier.

Social workers, because of their need to bring in partners within families, neighbourhoods and agencies to assist their service users and their carers, have strengths in communication and partnership working.

Because of the level of historical distrust which often exists within and between organisations, there is a need for courageous communication and co-working. Leadership has to be 'embodied'. As one commentator has argued:

> Our post-modern world makes it all the more important that we communicate with one another, build consensus, from a basis of strong conviction.

And again:

> This is about being visceral, passionate and embodied – speaking from the gut and the heart as well as from the head. For with this goes openness, honesty and earthiness.
>
> Webster, 2001: p3.

7. Planning, managing and deploying resources

The care management process, which we considered in Chapter 5, is an excellent micro-management system. Although many

---

Case Example 13

Barry, who had long-term enduring, and at times, acute paranoid schizophrenia, leading to a very chaotic lifestyle, had a poor relationship with his current care co-ordinator, erratic compliance with medication and viewed intervention as oppressive. His mental health deteriorated to a point where he was compulsorily admitted to hospital.

The medical and nursing views were that residential/nursing care was required at point of discharge. Following a social worker's assessment, it was felt that, although residential care would meet some of his needs, it would mean that he would have to give up his home, which he would find very difficult as he was attached to it – it was where his wife had died.

An alternative plan was sought which included seven-day home support, with support from a new care co-ordinator, who was a social worker. Barry was at first wary, but over time, established a trusting relationship. His previous problems of being exploited, poor financial management and therefore financial stresses, and having an insufficient diet were addressed, thus managing the stressors which had significantly impacted on his mental well-being.

Barry's views of the mental health services has now changed, to one of partnership, and he readily agrees to continue taking medication, thus assisting his continued residence in his own home attending community resources.

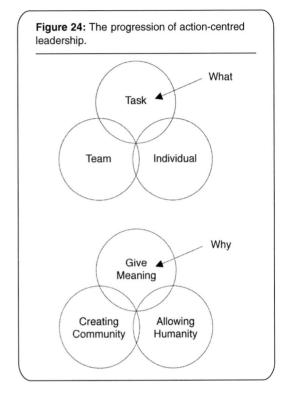

Figure 24: The progression of action-centred leadership.

- Clear and credible leadership with visible and active support of senior managers.
- A known and understood joint vision.
- Engagement in focused planning and implementation structures which include representation from all stakeholders.
- Addressing basic management issues in joint services such as conditions of service and line management and supervisory arrangements.
- Effective representation of wider social services responsibilities in planning (particularly childcare responsibilities).
- Application of performance management regimes.
- Services and care practice which place service users at their centre and which promote independence.
- Valuing diversity (particularly promoting culturally competent services).
- Robust and evidence-based approaches to risk assessment and management.
- A commissioning approach applied to all relevant services.
- Clear responsibility for co-ordinated care arrangements and a 'Whole System' approach which is performance managed.

From SSI, *Modernising Mental Health Services*, June 2002: p5.

social workers were resistant to care management as a concept, for many of the same reasons as a number of GPs were resistant to fund holding, i.e. that the management of a budget could constrain their assessment of need and mean a battle for the appropriate resources.

Whatever the ins and outs of the ethical dilemmas, however, care managers have to plan efficiently, deploy resources economically, and manage and evaluate the care package effectively, (see Figure 17).

Factors found to promote modernisation:

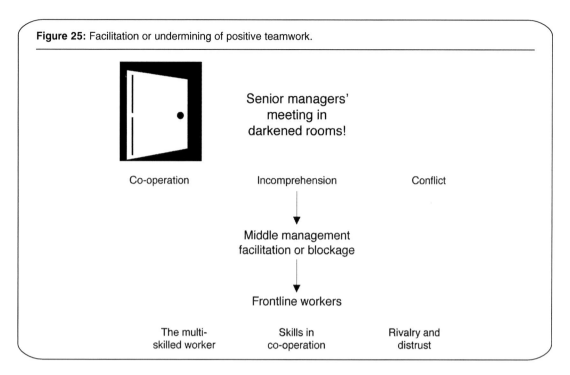

Figure 25: Facilitation or undermining of positive teamwork.

8. *Empowerment and accountability*

Thurstine Basset, one of my many very helpful correspondents while writing this book, mused that one of the paradoxes of being a member of a profession with an accent on facilitating, enabling and empowering is that it is difficult to broadcast success:

> *It is hard to point out the positive contribution when the contribution is centred on empowering others.*
> conversation with the author,
> 13th February 2002.

This empowerment, however, has to be a clear part of the management role. Delivering services to people through people, especially in a diversity of settings, cannot be done in a command and control manner. People have to be orientated, educated, trained and supported to work independently to promote people's independence.

Accountability is a matter for the manager and for the staff member jointly. Devolvement of responsibility by managers at any level must never be a shelving or shirking of responsibility. Devolution is not about abrogating responsibility.

Managers also need to role model 'followership' as well as 'leadership' (see Robert E. Kelley, November 1988). Good leaders demonstrate that they can follow as well as lead, and Martin Brown, who oversaw the introduction of the NSF for Mental Health, and is now Chief Executive of the Northern Development Centre for Mental Health, gives as a prime bit of career advice: 'First learn to follow before you aspire to lead' (quoted in *Health Service Journal*, 18th July, 2002).

9. *Building enduring organisations*

One of the factors which strikes one from the Westminster Study, which I've used extensively in this book, is that of the sheer 'stickability' of social workers in the face of extreme deprivation and distress. Organisations require stickability as well, and too often in the public sector there is a sense of panic if things don't appear to be going according to plan, and long-term corporate health is sacrificed for short-term gains.

Again, to quote from the commercial sector, Collins and Porras demonstrate that companies who have survived and generated enduring success have not necessarily been consistently successful:

'Indeed, all of the visionary companies in our study faced setbacks and made mistakes at some point during their lives, and some are experiencing difficulty as we write this book. Yet – and this is a key point – visionary companies display a remarkable *resiliency*, an ability to bounce back from adversity' (p4).

Public sector organisations particularly should take note of Collins and Porass' dictum that while strategies and tactics have to change to meet changing circumstances in a fast-changing world, core values should remain a constant.

Conclusion

Sometimes images and stories can be most effective in portraying what practice and management is about.

> *It's only a story, you say. So it is, and the rest of life with it . . . I can change the story. I am the story.*
> Jeannette Winterson, *The Power Book.*

Recently, a colleague of mine went white water rafting in America, and compared the experience to being a frontline manager in today's public sector organisations.

So to use this image, as a leader, at any level we have to:

- Set the direction in which we want to steer.
- Have expertise in negotiating both the surface water **and** the undercurrents.
- Have the ability to motivate and support the crew (as a group and as individuals) even when they are exhausted.
- Be able to negotiate obstacles.
- Work with people, not against them.
- Ensure that the boat is supplied with essential resources.
- Have the determination to complete the task.

Ours is overwhelmingly an individualistic society, but leaders have to be imbued with ideas of community and connection. We have to know ourselves, we have to lead ourselves, we have to be grounded in the present and be able to look to the horizon of the future; to take people with us we must convey a message and a meaning. **Ultimately we have to serve to lead.**

Chapter 8

Looking to the Future

Well, of course, I am still quite depressed and feel awful at times but I know that if things go wrong I can rely on my social worker. Out of all the people involved in my case, it is the social worker who is the best.

user quoted in SSI (2002) *Modernising Mental Health Services*, p12.

With new arrangements being put in place, often within health service structures, for the delivery of mental health services, it is increasingly important that the continuing contribution of social care perspectives and practitioners is recognised. Social care has an increasing track record of working in partnership with service users, and their carers and supporters, of commissioning services from a wide range of service providers, of developing practice and its management on the evidence-base, and of bringing a concern about the social context to the assessment and therapeutic processes. As new integrated organisational arrangements are established, valuing the strengths of social care becomes even more important.

Dr Ray Jones, former Chief Executive, Social Care Institute for Excellence, DSS, Wiltshire CC.

If you do not know which port you are sailing to, no wind is favourable.

Seneca, Roman philosopher.

We need to advocate for social work and social care, and we need to see the commissioning of social work and social care within a democratic framework.

David Behan, Director of Social Services for Greenwich and 2002/3 President of the ADSS.

While concentrating appropriately on the NSF, what were missing were a whole systems approach and an understanding of the complex nature of the mental health services arena.

SSI, op. cit. p46.

Social work, unlike other disciplines, does not have a tradition of relying upon consulting rooms or physically invasive intervention. The easy chairs, the pills and the needles have not been there as a signifier that something is being done to the mental health service user. This is a significant issue for people from black and minority ethnic groups. The feeling of being 'subjected to' something or someone undermines the experience of black and minority ethnic mental health service users, who collectively have a history of being in that position. Social work offers interventions based significantly on building a relationship with the service user in a physical and psychological context of empowerment. Social work offers a mechanism for building trust with those who receive cues from society and

from within mental health services, that institutions must not be trusted.

former SSI inspector and currently social care director of a mental health trust.

The necessity for social work

The irony of the current position is that social circumstances would seem to make the need for social work even more evident and imperative, and yet social work, at least in its current form and host organisation is often looked at askance. My philosophical eldest daughter once remarked in some perplexity, following changes at her primary school, that: 'nothing ever happens until it's actually happened'! And it must feel like this for many social work and social care staff who are being pulled in different directions, and may experience what Sir Roy Griffiths once remarked about community care that it is 'a poor relation; everybody's distant relative but nobody's baby', (Griffiths, 1988).

As the most recent publication on mental health policy asserts: 'Mental health and well-being are issues of everyday life and should be of interest to every citizen and employer, in addition to all care, education and administration sectors. Mental health is influenced (enhanced or jeopardised) in families and schools, on the streets and in workplaces – where people can feel safe, respected, included and able to participate, or maybe in fear, marginalised or excluded' (Jenkins et al., 2002: p3).

All the evidence from user research demonstrates a requirement to meet people's emotional and practical needs in a human way, and that a purely 'psychiatric response', as Cliff Prior, Chief Executive of Mental Health Charity Rethink (formerly the National Schizophrenia Fellowship) calls it (*Guardian Society*, 3rd July 2002: p11) often institutionalises people almost as thoroughly as the old mental hospitals.

It is important that the old debates between medical and social care approaches are not allowed to damage genuine attempts to provide services which are more flexible, responsive and accountable. Social care complements health intervention by ensuring that social experiences are considered and dealt with – such factors as racism, sexism, unemployment, difficulties in personal relationships, are key to the overall well-being of

the individual. Social care has a great deal to be proud of in having brought these issues to prominence.
                              social services director.

Kathleen Jones in her seminal history of mental health services charts a thematic wave of trends – a series of overlapping circles that progress with recurrent themes and challenges. Jones (Jones, K., 1972) saw the 1890 Act as 'the triumph of legalism', and following that a build up towards a more medical and treatment-orientated approach. 'It is only now', at her time of writing in the early 1970s, 'when the social services have developed a comparable professional status, which the social approach is coming into its own again', (p153). Ironically, it may be that the social approach is arriving sans social workers?! Denise Platt, Chief Inspector of Social Services, in an address to the National Institute for Social Work, expressed her concerns thus: 'I think social work is becoming a lost art – not to practitioners but to organisations, and as we lose it we realise what a contribution it has made'.

It is certainly clear to me that the social perspective, social work and social care are even more important now than they were. When social work commenced, with its roots in the 19th century, and grew through campaigners such as Mary Stewart, in the London Hospitals, where they refused to be boxed into a purely individualistic approach but insisted on reaching out to the community and seeing people in a holistic and whole systems way. Modern society is much more complex and deprivation increasingly visible. Despite strenuous efforts by Government, a number of social think tanks are indicating widening gaps between rich and poor in terms of health, housing, income, pensions etc. England is now no longer considered purely in terms of historical comparators, but as against Scotland, with its very different approach to some aspects of social welfare, and the continent as a whole (see Woodward and Kohli, 2001).

With the decline in feelings of solidarity with and responsibility for our fellow citizens; the removal of many effective powers from local authorities, and the building up of what Simon Jenkins calls 'the new magistracy' (see Jenkins, 1995), many people are increasingly excluded, and have difficulty in finding recourse. 'Modernism' with its often over-weaning optimism, has given place to 'post modernism' where 'we are our own little story-tellers, living

among the ruins of our former grand narratives', (Harvey, 1990). This may be fine if our innate sense of self is strong and we have confidence in our own stories, not so promising for those who have become lost and detached from their own inner reality and from other people.

Mental distress may be caused or compounded by poor living conditions and difficult personal circumstances. The role played by social workers can therefore be crucial to recovery from mental illness precisely because their focus is personal, giving practical support and help to resolve problems of living that might otherwise appear insurmountable to someone who is also trying to deal with his/her mental distress. This type of support not only contributes to recovery from a period of illness, it can also help to reduce the likelihood of a further episode recurring.
                  Michelle Rowett, Chief Executive,
                  Manic Depression Fellowship.

The situation for people from black and ethnic minority communities is particularly acute, as made clear by the statistics in earlier chapters of the book. The Sainsbury Centre's recent review of the relationship between Mental Health Services and African and Caribbean communities, *Breaking the Circles of Fear* (SCMH, 2002) speaks of services that fail to match the needs and aspirations of users and their families. Within all of this, 'culture is an important but much misunderstood and complex entity' (p64) and it is clear that the social work perspective of understanding somebody as an individual, but within their cultural and community context, but existentially again as an individual in their own right, is absolutely vital.

One of the National Institute for Mental Health in England's first national programmes is on 'Equalities', around issues of citizenship and social inclusion (see NIMHE, 2002 and Morris, 2001). Users of mental health services do not wish and see no reason why they should accept a concept where they are citizens one minute, and then, when they experience a mental illness, unlike those undergoing a physical ailment, are apparently removed from the society of citizens.

Users wish to be treated as fellow citizens, worked with in a human and empowering way; have their emotional and practical needs taken seriously and addressed; and given hope for the future.

Too many people have been allowed to sink into a chronic state, and as Topor asserts:

The cause of chronicity, which has long been sought within the individual (biological or psychological characteristics) is not inherent in the illness itself, a part of the natural order, but rather is clearly connected with the person's life in society.

Topor, 2000.

While fully acknowledging the strengths, expertise and courage of other professions, it has often struck me during my time as a practitioner and manager that it is social workers and social care workers who are willing, and adept at hanging onto the coat tails of the most deprived service users facing the greatest social dislocation. As society faces a number of dangerous fissures and fractures, like a land beset with earth tremors, it is the social worker who grapples with the whole picture. George O'Neill's fascinating study of role differentiation between CPNs and Mental Health social workers, points to the primary focus of CPNs on the individual, and the social worker on the individual and their systems (see O'Neill, 1997).

Just as it is dangerous to view people from ethnic minorities as of a homogeneous group, it is equally so with carers, as Michael Bainbridge demonstrates in a recent article for *Mental Health Today*, where he sees 'friends and families as innocent secondary victims of illness (the 'Medical Model'), where they are relegated to an entirely tangential role' (Bainbridge, 2002: p24). People are not just their caring role, but are individuals in their own right. It is perhaps significant that legislation around carers has placed duties on local authorities in an entirely appropriate way, and this is not the only thrust of government policy which implicitly or explicitly stresses the need for skilled social work interventions.

The Mental Health Act Commission in its latest biennial report (Mental Health Act Commission, 2001) and the comments of Margaret Clayton, the Chairperson, regarding the role of the approved social worker, has made it very clear about the value placed on the social work role and specifically that of the approved social worker. In fact, Clayton in her recent statement has said that:

The criteria for the Approved Mental Health Professional must be clearly set out so that they add to the value that Approved Social Workers currently do.
Community Care, 22nd August, 2002.

The small handbook on mental health social work produced by Oldham Social Services and Oldham NHS Trust describes the range of connections which social work makes.

Within the text, the authors make clear that:

Unchecked, the impact of a serious mental health problem will be very destructive of a person's quality of life. It often results in self-neglect, poverty ('social drift'), social isolation, social exclusion (including institutionalisation), depression and suicide. Mental Health social workers aim to work with individuals, carers, families, social groups and other related professions to counter these effects and to promote a greater sense of well-being, value and social inclusion.

p7.

Modernising Mental Health Services – the SSI Report

In June 2002, the SSI published its findings of its national survey of 19 authorities across six regions in England. In many ways the report is positive:

Much direct work with service users was valued by them. This was particularly true where work recognised their abilities as well as their needs and where it acted as a lifeline at a time of difficulty and as a passport to a range of helpful services.

In all councils, most service users expressed generally positive levels of satisfaction with the way that they were treated by staff. There were also examples of innovative services which promoted independence and positive lifestyles. These were particularly valued by users.

SSI, 2002: p1.

There were also, however, a number of cautionary signs:

- Good practice was often 'the result of past opportunistic development . . . stimulated and maintained by local champions', rather than it being the result of a more strategic approach.
- There was an insufficient strategic and practice link between mental health and children's services. This was being exacerbated in certain circumstances where structural change had seen a separation out of services for children from the traditional social services departments, and likewise mental health workers from social services transferring into mental health trusts.
- Black and minority ethnic communities were not well served even in 'councils with a robust general approach to equality issues, mental health services performance was poor' and this was especially true in joint services where the SSI 'found that there was an informal 'division of labour' under which

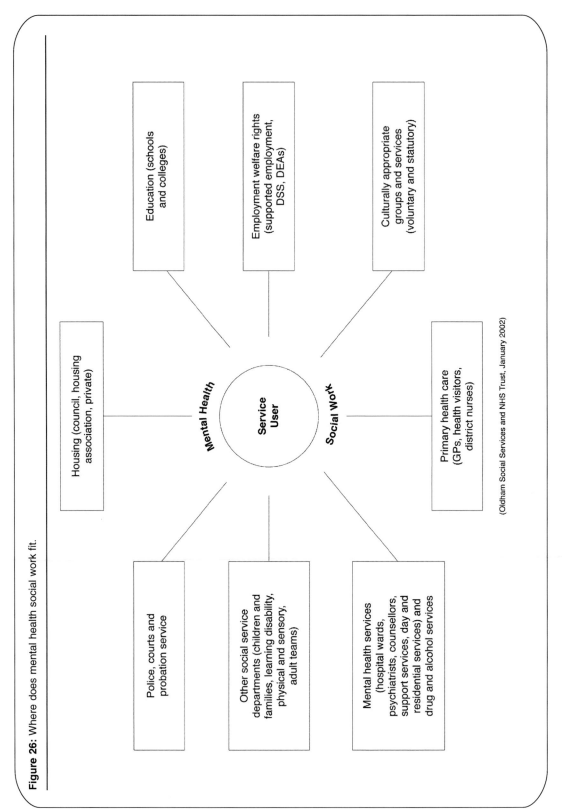

(Oldham Social Services and NHS Trust, January 2002)

Figure 26: Where does mental health social work fit.

equality and diversity issues were regarded as being the business of social services and not of the service as a whole' (p24).

Sadly, I've sometimes found component parts of the NHS have struggled with issues around user and carer involvement and promoting culturally competent services. It is something that social services staff working with or transferred into trusts can bring considerable expertise.

- The CPA was not always as user-focused as it could be. Common problems included:
  - Viewing the CPA as a review mechanism rather than as a systematic approach to identification and meeting of needs.
  - Not placing the service user at the centre of arrangements for their care.
  - Lack of attention to diversity issues.
  - Failing to address the needs of children and carers.
- Changes in structures were clearly major issues, and recent structural change, the lack of common boundaries, and a history of poor partnership arrangements clearly reflected in worse outcomes for users and carers.
- Social care needed a clear 'champion' within the system.
- Focus on the National Service Framework was essential, but so also was attention to the wider policy context.

A social care perspective adds significantly not just to the direct provision of services but to the strategic approach adopted within mental health services by taking this beyond a narrow focus on assessment and treatment of individuals.
　　　　　　　NIMHE Development Centre Director.

Change is not necessarily loss

I came into social work three years after Seebohm, and its introduction of social services departments, and the apparent misunderstanding that Seebohm's recommendation of the generic departments meant having generic workers.

It is easy to romanticise the past. The passing of the old mental welfare officer was much lamented, but picking up a number of cases from them in the early 1970s some people had clearly been offered routine monitoring rather than assessment and intervention suited to their specific needs.

In the 1990s the advent of care management was seen by many as an undermining of traditional social work, but where it was allied

to traditional social work values and skills, there were often benefits for service users and carers in procuring more personalised services.

The move towards care management as a function, and the continuing financial and demand pressures on Social Services meant that in many places the creative community role of social work was largely lost, to the extent that in a recent lecture David Morris, leading NIMHE's programme on equalities, has stated that other professions are moving into the gap that social work has left.

When we are educating and training social workers we are endeavouring to equip them with knowledge and understanding of a range of theories and perspectives, all of which will be relevant to their work in mental health settings. This includes professional perspectives, which will help them to work effectively in multi-disciplinary teams. It includes a wide range of theories, e.g. medical models of mental illness so that, although social workers may not use these models in their approach to their work, they can understand what they are and how to recognise them. It also includes service user perspectives, which will help them to become fully conversant with issues of diversity and inequality in relation to the provision of services.
　　　　　　　　　　　social work educator.

When I am not feeling defensive about my age I sometimes admit to having been a generic social worker! The value of course of the generic approach was its breadth, and the ability to transfer knowledge across the client groups and age ranges; the disadvantage, of course, was that it was just too broad and it was very difficult to attain and retain specialist knowledge across such diverse groups, and I must admit that I personally found it a relief to specialise in mental health and learning disability in the 1980s, though generic training and practice was extremely helpful when my management remit broadened in the 1990s. Specialisation has brought greater job satisfaction to social workers and increased appreciation of their work in specialist fields, but organisations such as Young Minds have expressed concern about the 'general level of awareness amongst social workers of mental health problems as they manifest themselves in children and young people, as well as a lack of awareness of prevalences', while acknowledging that there are 'outstanding examples of where . . . social workers are highly skilled in working with the psychodynamics of families and children', (conversation with the author, April 2002).

In 1982, the Barclay Report argued for a greater community focus for social work, while one of the minority reports by Professor Pinker argued strongly for a focus on a professional and statutory approach. The imperatives of work with people with mental health needs are for attention to both perspectives.

New organisations

There are clearly considerable merits in the formation of specialist Mental Health Trusts, especially in their ability to provide a co-ordinated service to users and carers, with the right skill mix of staff, and economies of scale. The caveats are also obvious:

- The new trusts must avoid the isolation from the broader aspects of mental health policy and practice. The SSI report of June 2002 raises some warning notes similar to the issues Kathleen Jones identifies in her studies of institutional approaches in her historical sweep of mental health services.
- There are concerns that the medical model may re-exert its dominance, though there are also hopes that the new structures will actually assist a social and environmental perspective.
- It is vitally important that primary care and secondary care are closely aligned and interlinked. The necessity for the long-term health of the organisation in involving users, carers and minority groups, and involving frontline staff must be really internalised in the NHS mindset.

I have remarked earlier about the tendency to seek structural solutions to complex challenges. The Northern Ireland model of integrated health and social care is often held up as a shining example, but Terry Bamford, who has managed services in both Northern Ireland and England at a Chief Officer level has warned about a too sanguine look across the Irish Sea (Bamford, 2000). Gulliver, Peck and Towell's study of The Somerset Integrated Approach, is clearly saying that the case for such change shows promise but is not yet proven (Gulliver, Peck and Towell, 2002) and increasing number of studies of change management in the private and public sectors counsel caution in instituting major structural change unless the arguments for such change are overwhelming.

During structural change, people inevitably turn inwards, worry about their own positions, lose contact with some of their networks which

bring about positive outcomes for users and carers, and suffer stress and exhaustion. Liam Hughes, a former Director of Social Services for Bradford and now Chief Executive of one of the Leeds primary care trusts, in a mainly positive article about change (Hughes, 2001, in Allen 2001) quotes Burke and Cooper (2000) who identify a range of dysfunctional reactions to change which is not well managed.

Hughes goes on to say that in many cases 'organisational memory has been lost and employees find it difficult to get their bearing. Loyalty is undermined, and pride diminished. These organisations have become unhealthy and anxious places' (Hughes, 2001: p74).

On the other hand, companies that do better have taken time to:

- Align and affirm their core values.
- Over-manage change.
- Communicate with and involve internal (staff) and external partners as much as possible.

Health and social care have operated under separate management and spending systems since the 1970s, but with increasing recognition that working collaboratively, both informally and formally, improves patient care. The initial mutual suspicions have given way to a mutual recognition of the value of the joint approach. It is particularly encouraging that most health care professionals now more than acknowledge the value of the skills of social care staff and have come to understand that the social model of care, with its emphasis on the individual, and daily living skills, enable people to achieve a better quality of life. The integration of health and social care is the last major barrier to bring down and should bring about major change for the better.

project manager, NIMHE Development Centre.

When I went to Staffordshire in 1992 as Operations Director, Adult Services, the imperative to bring in the National Health Service and Community Care Act into operation for the 1st April 1993, was one of the strongest challenges I have ever experienced. While meeting practical targets at all points, the team also desired to bring about a wider cultural change, and effected this by building on an initial change process over the next five years. I have met managers who genuinely believe that they have brought in much more far reaching changes than are evident, and this is because the ground is not laid for long-term, but is like a landscape hastily prepared, washed away by the first heavy rain. I have recently been working on a ten stage change process, building on John Kotter's work and that of Ann Proehl.

Successful leadership in multi-disciplinary settings requires:

- An understanding of a variety of perspectives and an ability to shape these to the needs of the service.
- Cultural sensitivity.
- An understanding of professional expertise and sensitivities, and an ability to align these with the good of the service, not to the narrow dictates of any one profession.
- Making the best use of the skill mix.
- Ensuring that all channels of communication are functioning.
- Ensuring that a whole systems approach is created and maintained.

Bob Hudson, from the Nuffield Institute, who has been researching the Health Act's flexibilities, concluded in a recent article (Hudson, 2002) that it was unclear where the care trusts constitute an answer to the causes of fragmented service delivery:

> *The fixation with structure has led to a preoccupation with the **means** of integrated working, and a neglect of the **ends**. Organisational change is only a proxy for the achievement of better outcomes ... The best way the debate can progress' is to have more emphasis 'on definitions of quality of life from the perspective of individual service users and their carers.*
>
> p10.

New professionals

George Bernard Shaw once said: 'All professions are a conspiracy against the laity', and we know in our hearts that there's a great deal of truth in this. The challenge is to become as professional, in the best sense, as possible while not building up the boundary fences which are so forbidding to users and carers.

Tony Russell, NIMHE Core Group colleague and user champion has always argued forcefully for a uni-professional approach so as to break down boundaries and increase co-ordination and the strength of relationship between professional and user. As a champion for the STR worker (Support, Time and Recovery) Tony is clear that this development comes from what users want.

On the other hand, other people I have spoken to believe it important to have the different perspectives, education and expertise of a range of professionals, especially those that counterbalance a biochemical approach where that is dominant. My own view is that it would

be unwise at this stage to attempt to merge all the professions. What should be happening is a focus on better outcomes for users, and a non-defensive approach by professions as to who is the best person to assist in achieving those outcomes at any one time. My own experience of working in a multi-disciplinary team in the 1980s is that this is perfectly possible. It is usually inadequate leadership and professional insecurity which leads to inappropriate professional defensiveness. Multi-disciplinary working, with the appropriate use of well-orientated and skilled support workers can provide a rich mix of skills which gives the service user and their carers more choice and access to a range of expertise.

As the above case study demonstrates, in well functioning teams, perspectives and skills are being shared, so that it is not always obvious who is a community nurse, an occupational therapist (as in the example above), a social worker, psychologist, psychiatrist etc. In the multi-disciplinary team I worked in people were confident in their professional identity and became increasingly confident and competent in their team identity. Professionalism was sought and attained but not used as a mask to blank out those we were working with, either users, carers or members of the public. Hughes calls this 'an identity of interest' (Hughes, 2001: p75). He points to new professions emerging as alliances grow, with some new features e.g.:

- Dual qualifications becoming more common, especially in mental health and learning disability.
- The possibility of a new profession around the assessment, care management and rehabilitation of older people, including those with mental health needs.
- New professions gradually emerging out of the new team services such as YOTs, Sure Start, regulatory services etc.
- The establishment of Connexions building bridges between careers, youth work, education, social work, residential work and after care.

Organisations and professions have an inbuilt tendency to serve their own internal needs. This is no longer acceptable.

The hidden social worker

One of my correspondents during this project, Thurstine Bassett, raised the interesting concept

Case Example 14

Success in the last chance saloon

A young Asian woman diagnosed with schizophrenia was on the verge of losing her 'last chance' place in a residential unit. Then Marianne Thomas and her team stepped in at the 11th hour to give her more autonomy – and keep her out of hospital

Case notes

Practitioner: Marianne Thomas

Field: Occupational therapist and outreach worker, assertive outreach team, mental health

Location: London

Client: Kashmira Narayan (not her real name) is a 24-year-old Asian woman who has been known to social services for seven years and has a diagnosis of schizophrenia. She also has a history of substance misuse, particularly solvents but other soft drugs also. She has been sectioned on several occasions.

Case History: Four years ago, following another spell under section in hospital, Narayan's family took her back to India to be married – hoping this would cure her illness. It made matters worse. Within months she returned to England without her husband, now estranged, because she was so unwell. She moved back in with her parents but this soon became untenable. The house was overcrowded, added to which Narayan's father, who drank excessively, was verbally and physically abusive towards her. A number of residential placements subsequently failed because Narayan was very chaotic, difficult to engage and challenging, while her solvent misuse escalated, endangering her health. She was also being exploited by a succession of boyfriends.

Dilemma: Narayan, a bright and articulate young woman, was proving very vulnerable to sexual and financial exploitation.

Risk factor: Supporting Narayan to become more independent may lead to more failure and see her sectioned again.

Outcome: Narayan is making slow but sure progress in taking control of her life.

Nine months ago a young Asian woman's hopes of getting a flat or a job seemed a lifetime away. Kashmira Narayan (not her real name), diagnosed with schizophrenia, was challenging her health and social care services to the limit. Already sectioned a number of times, there were serious doubt as that she could function healthily in the community. A challenging behaviour unit was emerging as the final option.

On the verge of having her last-chance residential care placement terminated, Narayan received a boost following the creation of a new assertive outreach team. With promised intensive support from the team, the residential home agreed to Narayan staying.

'While an in-patient she was aggressive and verbally abusive,' says outreach worker Marianne Thomas, who began working closely with Narayan. 'When we got to know her, a lot of the outbursts in the ward seemed part of a negative cycle. She'd have leave, would have an outburst, have leave stopped and so on.'

There was also concern about her solvent misuse and that she took cannabis regularly. 'This meant she felt that she was being locked up as 'a naughty girl', and felt she was being punished,' adds Jo Fuller, the assertive outreach team manager. It was explained to Narayan that although she might think that cannabis-taking was part of a 24-year-old's lifestyle, it has a negative effect on her condition.

'Because she felt she was in what seemed to her like prison,' adds Thomas, 'she was reacting to that. We saw our role as focusing on her as a person.' It was a focus that began to change her life. Although looking long-term, Thomas concentrated on getting Narayan established away from hospital and into the residential unit.

'We knew it could all go wrong,' says Fuller, 'but there really was something engaging about her.' Thomas agrees: 'There were a lot of practical things we could help with. She was very vulnerable. There was financial exploitation which was out of her control, which if eliminated would reduce the risk for her.'

Thomas arranged for Narayan's money to be managed by social services. 'She now gets an amount each day, which means that she doesn't have books that people can take and cash,' says Thomas. Although this action could be construed as controlling, Narayan agreed to it and is now relieved at the arrangement: 'It helped her realise what was happening. There was one person she was having a relationship with but who now doesn't want to see her because the money's not there.'

The outreach team work 365 days a year including weekday evenings, making themselves more available for Narayan. 'The big thing for her,' says Thomas, 'was seeing her as a person. Rather than focusing on 'are you taking your medication?' we'd go to the hairdressers or go swimming.' Realising that she can work with the team rather than kick against it, Narayan is responding well, particularly as she can see progress, albeit slowly, being made. 'She is attending an adult education class,' says Thomas, 'but still wants that normal life – that job, that flat. That's some way off but it seems a possibility now.'

Thomas, recognising Narayan's fractured relationships with family and boyfriends, focused on building trust. The 'everything up for negotiation' approach, belief in her possibilities for advancement, advocating on her behalf with other services ready to give up on her, and consistency in her life are delivering rewards. 'She's just asked if she can have a mobile phone,' smiles Thomas, 'so that when she's out or stays out she's able to keep in touch. Also she feels confident enough to tell us she's feeling unwell or hearing voices again – I think she knows that if she tells us things, we can work through it and stop her being sent back to hospital. So I think that trust is really working.'

'For years,' adds Fuller, 'she's either been in hospital and contained, or out and been completely chaotic. This is the first time she's been settled for years. And it can still all go wrong – she has a history of things going wrong, after all. But for every month that she's out and managing and coping, that's a positive thing – and all down to positive risk taking.'

For Narayan, having her own flat and a full-time job may still seem a lifetime away. But for now she's living safely in the community and Thomas is exploring the possibility of Narayan taking on some voluntary work for a couple of hours a week. It may be some years before there is light at the end of the tunnel – but at least they're in that tunnel and travelling the right way.

Arguments for risk
- The team were sure that with the right support it would be possible for Narayan to live in the community. Narayan deserved another chance to experience more independence and the improvement in the quality of life that goes with that.
- For the first time in years, Narayan was achieving some stability and building trust in her life and the time was right to make progress on that.
- Although Narayan argued cogently against nurse-injected medication to convince the team that she should use replacement oral medication, she has shown maturity by understanding that she needs some sort of medication and that if the new system fails to work she will resume with the injections.
- Narayan's residential home has worked well with the team despite ambivalence from some care staff about giving Narayan one more chance. This has provided a permanent base for her – adding to the consistency in her life.

Arguments against risk
- Narayan's recent history would indicate the possibility of misusing drugs again. The more she felt she was living a normal life, the more she might be tempted to take drugs – something she

considers part of a normal lifestyle. The scale of her solvent misuse had caused worries about possible brain damage, with cannabis also having a negative effect on her condition.
- As Narayan enjoys more independence, there is the possibility that she may cut off contact and revert to her old lifestyle. This may result in her being sectioned again.
- Given the team's open and non-restrictive approach to working with Narayan, she might consider that the team are condoning her actions.
- At her last care plan approach meeting it was agreed, although not without reservation, that rather than a nurse administered system, she would receive replacement oral medication, which, although managed by the staff in her care home, would give Narayan more opportunity to avoid taking it.

Independent comment
The family's arrangement to have Narayan return to India is a typical response when an individual presents delusional and bizarre behaviour, the belief being that local healers can erode the spirits that are causing the behaviour, writes Raj Jhamat. It is also a common response to have a woman married off without fully detailing her mental health difficulty to her future husband and in-laws. This more than often leads to young women being traumatised by abusive in-laws and subjected to domestic violence.

The support Narayan requires appears to have been identified in clinical terms but there is a missing element around independence. Within Asian communities, connections to family and the community are far stronger than those of the white population. Isolation can lead to further mental health difficulties.

At Sahayak befriending service in Kent, we offer support to people rebuilding lives outside of the family. We also seek to build bridges back to the community.

Mental health promotion helps families and community leaders understand the complexity of mental health difficulties and to remove taboos. Gaining the community leaders' support opens up referral channels that would otherwise avoid existing statutory services.

The complex difficulties facing Narayan must be faced by a multi-agency team approach along with support for the family, enabling her to feel secure in her rehabilitation.

Raj Jhamat is a National Schizophrenia Fellowship community mental health worker.

Reprinted by kind permission of *Community Care*, 21–27 March, 2002.

of 'the hidden social worker'. Some years ago it would have been unlikely to have seen anybody move from social work into a different organisational setting; chief executives of local authorities, for example, were almost all from a legal or financial background. Increasingly now, however, people with a social work background are becoming chief executives of Local Authorities, Mental Health Trusts, PCTs, moving into different aspects of government and related organisations such as the LGA.

It is to be hoped that social work with its perspective on the individual and on wider society will have something particular to add.

> There will be other storms to face. Social work is a difficult and complex task; we will never know enough, or have enough resources, or work for sufficiently competent organisations for the job always to be done as well as the client deserves and the social worker wishes. I do not expect social work to be popular. It deals with people society would usually prefer to forget; unwanted, stigmatised, dependent. It does not do so quietly, but acts as an irritant by standing up for their rights and needs.
> Sir William Utting, former Chief Social Work Officer, DHSS.

Possible pathways

> There is no linear evolution; there is only a circumambulation of the self.
> Carl Jung, *Memories, Dreams, Reflections.*

> We shall not cease from exploration
> And the end of all our exploring
> Will be to arrive where we started
> And to know the place for the first time.
> T. S. Eliot, *Little Giddings* (1888–1965).

Jane Lewis, in a recent collection of essays (Allen, 2001) remarks on the positive feelings amongst many social work and social care staff when they moved from a health-based organisation to the new social services departments in 1971. It should be said, however, that this was not a universal expression, many people from a mental health background who I met when I came into social services in 1974, were strongly of the opinion that being under the auspices of an able and energetic medical officer of health gave them an advantage in building up resources which looked at a whole community approach, and certainly when one looks at some of the outstanding medical officers of health, their concept of individual and public health and their mutual congruence were certainly influential in promoting approaches which we would now put under

headings such as social inclusion, health promotion etc. (See Dickens and Gilbert, 1979.)

Since 1971, organisational approaches have swayed this way and that, but some of the most productive for users and carers, and the most satisfying for social work staff and their colleagues in other disciplines, have been where social workers have worked in multi-disciplinary teams, but had strong links with their own profession. Part of the unease currently is to do with some aspects of organisational culture within the NHS – for example, one major trust being criticised by an inner CHI report for focusing on performance targets and its financial deficit rather than clinical governance, clinical outcomes and service planning. It is not reassuring to social work and social care staff to hear one of the apparently leading trusts in the country admitting that it needed 'to give clinical quality as much priority as money and activity'! (see *Health Service Journal*, 15th August 2002: p4). The possible resurgence and reassertion of a medical model is another cause for concern, and this is ironically more likely in Trusts, allied to medical schools, with a strong emphasis on medical leadership; so much depends on how psychiatry defines itself in the future and educates and trains its practitioners. Links back to the wider social work profession, local government and professional guidance are also crucial; a number of transfers of staff by Local Authorities do not appear to have effectively retained these links and this commissioning strength, so that staff feel effectively cut adrift.

> As a qualified social worker and now as Chief Executive of MIND, I know that social work has been key in developing a broader based and more holistic approach to mental health than was previously the case when it was exclusively in the hands of the medical profession.
> Richard Brook, Chief Executive, MIND.

Possible routes for social work could be:
1. Social workers as part of integrated teams in mental health trusts or care trusts.

This would be an extension of current trends under the Health Act flexibilities. The social work role remains substantially as it has been historically, but there are huge opportunities for enunciating and promoting social perspectives and the value-base of social work as a profession, while at the same time taking on board the perspectives, skills and values of other professions. Duncan Double, a consultant psychiatrist and honorary senior lecturer with the University of East Anglia, writes cogently of this kind of approach in a recent article (Double, 2002), and Martin Webber, a social worker/care manager in a community mental health team in the Borough of Kingston-upon-Thames, speaks of the 'invigorating' climate of working in a multi-disciplinary setting. (*The Independent*, 25th February 2002.)

Gulliver, Peck and Towell's warning in the light of their evaluation of the integration of health and social services in Somerset, is that a focus on structures as opposed to outcomes and how to ensure these, can lead to unreal and unrealised expectations, (Gulliver, Peck and Towell, June, 2002). These caveats around structural change are also there in the debate around the future shape of children's services. Jane Held, Co-chairperson of the ADSS Children and Families Committee, and Director of Camden Social Services cautioned that:

> . . . it is crucial to remember that child protection is at the centre of working with kids. It is also **everybody's responsibility**. If you separate it out and give it to a new agency, it becomes **somebody else's responsibility** and that magnifies rather than reduces risk.
>
> Community Care, 29th August, 2002.
> (my emphasis).

This will be a problem for the mental health trusts if they separate themselves from the wider social inclusion agenda and for local authorities if they fail to honour their commitment to mental health in all its manifestations.

> Social workers have contributed in many valuable ways to the development of Mental Health strategies in recent years, and we need to build on that resource.
>
> The Revd Dr Peter Sedgwick,
> Church of England,
> Board of Social Responsibility.

Social services departments will need to ensure that there is a champion for social work and social care within the new organisations, and proper commissioning and professional connections maintained and nurtured.

> There are generalised feelings being expressed that the role of social work and that of the Approved Social Worker is not understood or valued. This seems particularly highlighted when social workers are in teams where there is a manager from the Health Services rather from a social work background – though this is not always the case – much seems to depend on individual managers and their approach to and willingness to understand the social perspective and the role which social work can play.
>
> social work educator.

2. Part of a new unified profession.

The introduction of STR workers and other front-line workers, who will be alongside service users in the way that the latter have expressed a need for, and the many research studies across client groups which have shown an impatience and confusion with the range of different professionals entering people's homes, gives some indication that we may be moving towards a single profession. Certainly joint training courses are coming more into vogue, but in the past joint professional awards have not always been given the required recognition, and it is to be seen whether the new organisations are more forthcoming.

One concern would be that the new support workers could become over-professionalised and lose the 'whole person, whole life' approach that has been particularly appreciated by service users (see Smith, Professional Dilemma, *Community Care*, 11th April 2002). On the other hand, the different professions could lose something in their integration, and so could service users. In a conversation with a nurse manager recently, he told me 'I don't feel the fully generic worker will give the quality and range of experience and skills that users need', (conversation with the author, 2002). This was echoed in a conversation that I had with a social work team, who also felt that the particular professional training, skills and values which the different professions brought, properly co-ordinated, gave a greater richness to the service users and carers they served.

> The development of CMHTs, and the care programme approach in the last decade was pivotal in 'democratising' the professions in mental health, helped by the role of CMHT manager, which is often undertaken by someone with a social work training. This democratisation is now under threat as the trusts develop, the role of social worker is in real danger of being 'downgraded' and subsumed within the 'medical model' with health as the dominant partner.
>
> social work team leader.

3. Social workers in Primary Health Care Teams.

One of the most beneficial approaches in recent times has been the increasing propensity to place social workers in primary care settings. While this is no panacea, and resources and specialisation create a number of challenges, general practice/primary care is so crucial to the health of the majority of the population that better communication between the professions, increased access for users and carers, and a shared understanding of the benefits of different approaches and perspectives has produced better outcomes for all concerned.

I have already quoted the Worcestershire approach (Le Mesurier and Cumella, 2001), and recently the *Health Service Journal* carried an enlightening article around the approach in Hull (see Banyard et al., 2002: p24–5). In most inner cities, there is a heightened incidence of single-handed general practitioners, which creates additional challenges in terms of communication and resources. Many singleton GPs who I worked with as a practitioner, especially in my role as an ASW, were considerably more problematic to work with than those within a group practice. It is interesting that at least one single-handed GP in Hull is quoted as saying that having a social worker attached was 'like the light at the end of the tunnel'. One can see that the presence of GP attached social workers, alongside the advent of the new primary care workers, will bring increased benefits to the delivery of mental health services.

> *Ultimately, the great strength of social work as a subject area lies in the sheer scope of the knowledge and experiences it draws upon. But its great weakness also lies in this wide scope, because without careful articulation of its aims and purpose, and a selective approach to deciding which theories best meet these aims and objectives in practice in particular contexts, then social work can seem an ineffective approach to bringing about change in people's lives.*
> social work educator.

4. The role of the Approved Social Worker.

The role and practice of the ASW has been one of the enduring benefits of the 1983 Mental Health Act. Successive Mental Health Act Commission biennial reports and the findings of mental health enquiries have shown the value of these well trained practitioners with a holistic, individual and social systems approach.

While both BASW and the ADSS have accepted a need for change because of the shifting tectonic plates of society and organisations, all the relevant bodies and all professions see an essential need to carry forward the skills and perspective of the ASW into the new system. This has been most clearly articulated by Margaret Clayton, as Chairperson of the Mental Health Act Commission (see Clayton, 2002).

The British Association of Social Workers, in its response to the consultation on the Draft Mental Health Bill (BASW, September 2002) puts it:

> *It is essential that the official taking on the quasi-judicial element of the present ASW role should be trained to the same standard, should be capable of evaluating the social and environmental aspects of the case, and should above all be demonstrably independent of the health body which was proposing the use of compulsory powers.*
> p2.

Andrew McCulloch, formerly Director of Policy for the Sainsbury Centre for Mental Health, and now Chief Executive of the Mental Health Foundation, sees the demise of the ASW as a great loss to users and carers, the judicial system, multi-disciplinary perspectives and to the social work profession. The fact that this social work role was defined by statute, praised by independent bodies and colleagues, as well as users and carers, and had a link back with the wider local government agenda, is something that gave social work considerable credibility and prestige.

> *Approved social workers bring a healthy and independent view to the process of sectioning and compulsion. Indeed, I would welcome a strengthening and developing of this role. Approved social workers provide an essential buffer between psychiatrists and individuals at the point of using compulsory powers, as long as ASWs are able to retain their independence.*
> Richard Brook, Chief Executive, MIND.

The Mental Health Act Commission makes it clear that the ASW has a wider role than purely reacting to requests for admission to hospital (Mental Health Act Commission, 2001) and this is echoed in a recent article by Greg Slay, a Mental Health Practice Development Manager with West Sussex County Council, and a member of BASW's Mental Health Special Interest Group, when he says that 'ASWs also need to be supported and valued in developing that wider role by their employing authority' (Slay, July 2002).

One of the problems BASW sees with the current ASW role is, just as in the case in a great deal of statutory childcare work, ASWs are being pushed into an increasingly functional, though valuable, task and not able to perform their wider therapeutic functions. Dr Double, a consultant psychiatrist, who is part of the Critical Psychiatry Network, and a supporter of social perspectives, sees that there is a:

> *. . . case for arguing that such a move could free social workers from the bureaucracy and officialdom of the ASW role to use their knowledge and skills more broadly in working with users and their families,*

allowing them to return to their traditional emphasis on the social model.

Double, September, 2002.

5. A return to a community work model.

When I was practising as a generic social worker in the 1970s, our office had a community worker. The Barclay Report should have seen an extension of this community approach, but the pressures of statutory work have tended to diminish the availability of social workers to develop community resources.

The people who will need social care remain however the pieces are moved around the board to try and ensure the best possible delivery of services to them.

ADSS, Review of ADSS Needs, Structures and Resources, June 2002.

John Pierson's recent work (Pierson, 2002) demonstrates a need for social work and its current local authority host to rediscover this community dimension, and for social workers moving into Health and Social Care settings to promote this perspective. Unfortunately, the draft of the Mental Health Bill as at the time of writing has reduced the place of local authorities (e.g. the removal of a Section 117 duty) and so some of the social perspectives may be lost.

In all of this, social work needs to feel valued as it gives value to those it works with. The recent Audit Commission Report (*Recruitment and Retention*, September 2002) demonstrates starkly the workforce challenges and how critical a motivated workforce is 'to delivering the reform agenda and improvement of public services' the Government desires (the Audit Commission's Director for Public Services Research, quoted in *The Guardian*, 4th September 2002).

There is a concern that, at a time when social work is probably needed more than ever, it may be overtaken by events. No profession has an inherent right to survive, and while professionalism is always important, professions sometimes put up such walls around them that they are no longer permeable by outside influences, especially by those who use the service.

As a history graduate, I am always acutely aware of the issues around cultural identity and cultural transference. There is, for example, a theory that Anglo-Saxon culture flourished so quickly and profoundly because the Romano-Britons had been able to transfer their cultural achievements to social groups who brought a different, but also rich culture with them, leading to a new and creative cultural landscape. It may be that one of social work's major roles now is to carry the holistic and social perspectives into other settings and enriching those and other professions.

Power and empowerment

The love of liberty is the love of other people, the love of power is the love of ourselves.

William Hazlit (1778–1830).

Only connect . . . and human love will be seen at its highest. Live in fragments no longer.

E. M. Forster, Howard's End.

We need to work with clarity and pride with other professionals. After all, social workers are streets ahead with empowerment, advocacy and consultation, and participation with service users. Nowhere is a person-centred response more obvious . . . Surely as professionals, if we truly believe in what we are doing, we will continue to promote and demonstrate such principles.

Margaret Reed, social worker,
(quoted in Reed, April 2002).

In multi-disciplinary settings, power relationships are both explicit and opaque. Thompson pinpoints three levels – individual, cultural and structural – with power as the common factor (Thompson, 2001). Relations between users and carers and staff members, or the team as a whole, and relationships between teams, can become corrupted and pathological if there are individual power struggles, battles within discourse – language and culture; and class, gender and other structural conflicts.

Unless services are sensitive to power issues then certain groups can see themselves as not just outside an ostensibly helpful system but oppressed by it. This is demonstrated very graphically in the Sainsbury Centre's recent review of the relationship between mental health services and African and Caribbean communities, *Breaking the Circles of Fear* (SCMH, 2002), and issues for women (see e.g. Kohen, 2000). For some groups there are issues around double discrimination, e.g. for black women (see Chantler, 2002) older people, people with learning disabilities etc.

Health service professionals are often found, quite rightly, bemoaning the discrimination of people experiencing mental distress, by other members of the community. But professionals themselves put up 'them and us' barriers. Rachel Perkins, Clinical Director of Adult

Mental Health Services for the South West London and St George's Mental Health NHS Trust, writing from the perspective 'of both a provider and a recipient of mental health services', states that the first requirement of helping 'people rebuild their lives' is 'to be able to form relationships with our clients that foster and maintain hope'. To do this, professionals need to be able to:

- Value the person for who they are.
- Believe in their worth.
- Listen to and heed what they say.
- Believe in the authenticity of their experiences.
- Accept and actively explore these experiences.
- See and have confidence in their skills, abilities and potential.
- Tolerate uncertainty about the future.
- See problems and setbacks as part of the recovery process.

The next requirement is to help people to make sense of what has happened and in taking back control. This involves helping people to:

- Reach an understanding of what has happened to them that makes sense to them and allows the possibility of growth and development.
- Mobilise their internal resources, especially their confidence and self-belief, and recognise their skills and ambitions.
- Gain control over their problems and to decide what they want to do in their life.

The third aspect is to enable people to access the roles, relationships and activities that are important to them, and the resources and support they need to pursue them. This involves providing assistance and support to:

- Maintain existing activities and relationships.
- Reduce the barriers that prevent people from accessing new things they want to do, and gain access to the material resources and opportunities that are their right.

Perkins ends by saying that:

Most of all, practitioners must learn from those whom they serve ... Perhaps the real challenge is to move towards a position where we put our expertise at the disposal of service users, rather than making decisions for them and doing to them.

Perkins, September 2002.

An important and frequently very moving aspect of the user's voice is not uncommonly the experience of 'treatment' as some form of attack on the symptoms rather than assistance with the difficulties they are trying to negotiate. I am convinced that one of the reasons behind this disparity is a continuing failure to set patients' [sic] symptoms, difficulties and disabilities within their social context.

consultant psychiatrist.

So much of the underlying attribute of the 'skilled helper' is that of an ability to use professional authority where appropriate, but eschew the easy recourse to the use of power. The use of power can never be neutral, while one person accrues power to themselves they inevitably remove power from other people.

*For many black and minority ethnic mental health service users, a social worker represents a mental health professional who will reach out to build a relationship. The relationship is intended to ensure that the service user can get what they need (accommodation, benefits, work) rather than the social worker using the relationship to broker the right to do something to the service user. Black and minority ethnic people feel they have suffered too long at the hands of those determined to do things **to** them.*

SSI Inspector, now Director of Social Care for a Mental Health Trust.

I was struck, when reading Kay Redfield Jamison's autobiography, *An Unquiet Mind* (Jamison, 1995), how she describes her psychiatrist. Jamison herself is a professor of psychiatry at the John Hopkins University School of Medicine, and experienced bouts of extreme and life-threatening manic depression. Jamison is very frank about her fight against the taking of Lithium to control her bi-polar mood swings, a reluctance based on a number of considerations, all of which were understood by her psychiatrist but, as she describes him, he was:

Very tough, as well as very kind, and even though he understood much more than anyone how much I felt I was losing – in energy, vivacity and originality – by taking medication, he never was seduced into losing sight of the overall perspective of how costly, damaging, and life-threatening my illness was. He was at ease with ambiguity, had a comfort with complexity, and was able to be decisive in the midst of chaos and uncertainty. He treated me with respect, a decisive professionalism, with an unshakeable belief in my ability to get well, compete and make a difference.

Jamison, 1995: p88.

That ability to balance professionalism with the personal, complexity with a stable and clear-sighted view of the long-term goals, and authority without the abuse of power, is something that is absolutely vital for the practitioner and for the manager. As I said before, a great many of the issues for practitioners are also there for managers at whatever level. The latest work by Jim Collins (Collins, 2001) focuses on what he calls 'level 5' leadership, which is essentially about the humility of great leaders who channel their ego needs into the greater good of the organisation, rather than into their own ambitions.

It is sometimes easier to get at these issues through literature or film. For me, the American writer, Ursula Le Guin, has an amazing facility for describing and encapsulating the individual's need to leave the world a better place than when they found it, without abusing their gifts or position, and without encroaching on the life and liberty of other people inappropriately. In *The Lathe of Heaven*, George Orr's ability to dream different realities is manipulated by his therapist, Haber. Haber appears powerful but:

> The big man was like an onion, slip off layer after layer of personality, belief, response, infinitely as layers, no end to them, no centre to him. Nowhere that he ever stopped, had to stop, had to say here I stay! No being, only layers.
>
> Le Guin, 1971: p80.

Orr initially trusts Haber because he sees him as 'not an evil man. He means well', but what Orr objected to is Haber's 'using me as an instrument, a means – even if his ends are good' (p44). Orr begins to feel that the therapist is without a centre, without integrity 'The doctor was not, he thought, really sure that anyone else existed, and wanted to prove that they did by helping them'. (p27).

In the end, Haber takes over the dreaming from Orr, in order to accelerate the move towards a perfect world as Orr sees it. But because Orr has no core to his own being, his dreams, far from creating a new reality, completely undo any kind of reality, creating a world which is literally insane and unbound.

Likewise, in the Earthsea Quartet, in the third book, *The Farthest Shore*, the desire of one man who has had magical powers to do good, but has now abrogated to himself the ambition to cheat death, is draining all life and colour and energy from the world around him. When the hero, Ged, confronts the man who is now neither dead nor alive, he challenges him that he sold everything to save himself, but now 'you have no self. You have given everything for nothing'. To try and gain everything he has

created a nothingness, as did Haber with his empty dreams of ambition. Ged goes on to say:

> And so now you seek to draw the world to you, all that light and life you lost, to fill up your nothingness. But it cannot be filled. Not all the songs of earth, nor all the stars of heaven, could fill your emptiness.
>
> Penguin Books (Quartet Edition), 1993: p463.

When Ged asks the other man what life is, the other's response is 'power'; and again in the answer to 'what is love?' again, he gives the answer 'power'.

To close the door between the world of the dead and world of the living, and to make it whole again, Ged has to sacrifice all his own powers.

> Social workers, along with others, including service user groups, have been part of a strong coalition that has challenged traditional stereotypes in mental health. This has led to a greater emphasis on rights and more quality being seen in the relationships within mental health work as far as service users are concerned.
>
> Richard Brook, Chief Executive, MIND.

Such things are repeated in Le Guin's extraordinary study of individuals and social systems – *The Dispossessed*. The physicist, Shevek, lives on a world without any explicit power structures, part of a group of people who emigrated from the host world where Le Guin depicts capitalist and totalitarian systems. But the community set up without power structures has been corrupted by a group who suppress ideas by ignoring them, by refusing to think, refusing to change. As Shevek's friend points out, the person who is suppressing his radical ideas:

> . . . has power over you. Where does he get it from? Not from vested authority, there isn't any. Not from intellectual excellence, he hasn't any. He gets it from the innate cowardice of the average human mind. Public opinion! That's the power structure he's part of, and knows how to use. The unadmitted inadmissible government that rules the Odonian society by stifling the individual mind.
>
> Le Guin, 1974: p142.

Shevek faces this by undertaking a personal journey of self discovery and using his own centeredness and integrity as a way of making new connections with people and helping them to confront themselves, not always successfully. At the end, in a common theme for Le Guin, he returns to where he started. Like the social worker who uses their own integrity to get alongside other people in distress: 'he had not brought anything. His hands were empty, as they had always been' (p319).

Creating value

To a large extent, we're the keepers of each other's stories, and the shape of these stories has unfolded in part from our interwoven accounts. Human beings don't only search for meanings, they are themselves units of meaning; but we can mean something only within the fabric of larger significations.

Eva Hoffman, *Lost in Translation*, 1989: p279.

It is time for social work to recover its ambition as an organised and cohesive force for good in society.

Bill Utting, former Chief Inspector, SSI, June 2002.

I have striven not to laugh at human actions, not to weep at them, nor to hate them, but to understand them.

Benedict Spinoza, born 1632.

Everyone is interesting who will tell the truth about him (or her) self.

Quentin Crisp (quoted in Beresford) 2002.

Running a half marathon around Wolverhampton a few weeks ago, I got into a conversation with a fellow club member who is an engineer. 'I don't envy you guys,' he commented, 'we're both in the business of risk, but when I am considering the strength of steel, I know what pressure I can put it under, what weights and tensions it will bear, before it breaks. You are dealing with human beings, who knows when they will break, whether it's at the point of greatest pressure, or when the pressure has seemingly been removed, and then some small straw causes the human structure to fracture. And at the end of the day, if you choose to intervene or not to do so, you are open to blame and very little praise'. Just as mental distress and mental ill-health is something that needs to be experienced at some level to gain a real insight, though profound empathy can almost get there, so social work is a calling which needs to be experienced to gain an insight into its complexity. When I was a trainee social worker and social worker in an area office, we shadowed medical and nursing colleagues and the GP Trainee Scheme sent its doctors to shadow social services staff. This was enormously beneficial in long-term understanding and relationship building. I directly experienced lives being saved through the understanding that was built up at this level.

In a recent article in *Community Care* (7th March, 2002), a medical student shadowed social workers in Sheffield:

My view totally changed when I worked with social workers. I have a lot of respect for those doing the job.

It is not a 9–5 job – it offers a 24-hour 7-day-a-week service. It's hard to switch off from some of the stuff they deal with when they go home. It takes a certain type of person to do it. It certainly does!

All the evidence from research, from talking to users and carers, from reading autobiographies like Kay Redfield Jamison's tells us that people experiencing mental distress and mental illness, of whatever type, but especially that which is enduring and/or cyclical, requires people of great integrity, sensitivity, resilience, skill and 'stickability' to work with and stay with those who are in Swinton's words 'hanging on' (Swinton, 2001).

As one of the most pertinent research studies demonstrates (MacDonald and Sheldon, 1997: p. 51.): 'The role of specialist social workers was obviously pivotal in the system of care. They both arranged for services, and were a service *themselves*'. (An awkward principle for those who speak and write about 'services', as if these were always 'things'). In this study, the social services staff emerged as individuals to be relied upon to provide emotional support and counselling, for a range of practical services and for their well-respected 'advocacy' function. This appears to have been carried out with a distinctive friendliness, openness and professionalism which, for the majority of respondents, was thought to be the best thing about the help they received.

Professor Peter Beresford of Brunel University, who describes himself as a long-term user of mental health services, speaks of a need to focus on language and meaning; ourselves and our identities – keeping in touch with who we actually are; and between social settings and individuals, (Beresford, February 2002).

The language of distance, of dispossession, of dichotomy are well developed in our society. We prefer to talk about 'them' and 'us' rather than 'us' and 'us'. In a recent article in *The Observer*, (1st September 2002) on stress at work the author was very keen to emphasise that this was social distress and not mental distress, inviting us to think that if we suffer from mental distress, we don't need to identify with people who experience a mental illness. So much healthier are those people who took part in the recent exhibition where stories of well-known people exemplified the normality of moving through different states and stages of life. As Beresford puts it:

I am simply saying that if we start by seeking to understand and be honest about ourselves to ourselves, we may well be able to be more understanding and less judgemental of others and of madness and distress. What begins as a denial of who we are ends up as a denial of the rights of others to be who they are, just as surely as what begins as the burning of books ends with the burning of people. We must start with ourselves.

Beresford, February 2002: p29.

It is social work and social workers who are at the margins, walking the boundaries of the forgotten lands with forgotten people; raising their voices for the dispossessed; valuing the unvalued; combating stigma for those we stigmatise; working to empower those who are disempowered. The philosopher, William James, once wrote that he had 'done with great things and big things, great institutions and big successes, and I am for those tiny invisible molecular moral forces that work from individual to individual, creeping through the crannies of the world like so many rootlets, or like the capillary oozing of water . . .' Social work works to empower and transform (see Payne, 2002), and fight for justice for individuals and social justice; and this is especially pertinent in the role of the approved social worker and the area where the individual collides with the law.

Social workers have been part of the recognition that Mental Health is not just about hospital and medication but about care, support, rights and opportunities, to be citizens on an equal basis.

Richard Brook, Chief Executive of MIND.

Social work is about recognising the individuality and innate dignity of each person, connecting with them, seeing the whole person in the context of their past and future aspirations, their family and neighbourhood, their community and connections. It is about building on integrity and creating trust and meaning, listening to and walking with, comprehending culture, race and creed, and engaging with the lived experience.

We are all complex individuals, living in a complex world. This complexity requires a response which is both direct and sophisticated. These skills are even more imperative today when we seem to be, like Ernest Shackleton and his team of Antarctic explorers, sailing out into the unknown and striding along uncharted shores. The historian, David Cannadine (Cannadine, 2002) speaks of a history of economics and sociology, of causes and explanation, developing into a history of psychology and anthropology, a cultural approach to history around meaning and understanding. Patricia Shaw in her *Changing Conversations in Organisations* (Shaw, 2002) speaks of horizons being so complex that 'we must recognise that we are shaping the evolving meaning of living experience as an ongoing creative social endeavour. Our present sense-making acts back to reshape the meaning of the past which changes the possible meaning of the future – lively enquiry amidst diversity is key. We can never be in control and need to rethink what it means to be in charge' (Shaw, lecture to the ADSS Spring Seminar, 2002, see also Parton and O'Byrne, 2000: Chap 1).

When one looks at Daniel Goleman's work on leadership, one sees that his components of emotional intelligence at work: self-awareness, self-regulation, motivation, empathy and social skill (Goleman, 1998) speaks very much to what social work is about. We are all explorers now of meaning, of diversity and identity, of boundaries, of hope and aspiration.

As one service user put it 'My social worker picked up that I was ready to explore sort of what was happening to me' (quoted in *Mental Health Foundation*, 2002).

We don't yet know the future for social work, so in the words of Dag Hammarskjold 'For all that has been – thanks, for all that will be yes' (*Markings*, Faber and Faber, 1964).

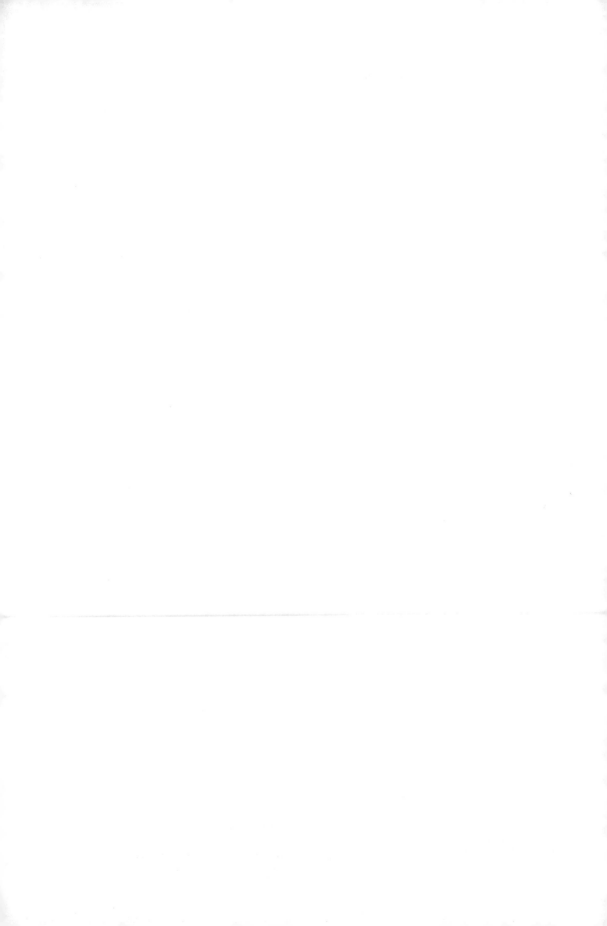

References and Further Reading

Adair, J. (1973) *Action-Centred Leadership*. London, McGraw-Hill.

Adair, J. (1983) *Effective Leadership*. Aldershot, Gower.

Adair, J. (1987) *Effective Teambuilding*. London, Pan.

Allen, I. (Ed.) (2001) *Social Care and Health: A New Deal?* London, Policy Studies Institute/University of Westminster.

Allott, P. and Loganathan, L. (2002) *Discovering Hope for Recovery from a British Perspective: A Review of a Sample of Recovery Literature, Implications for Practice and Systems Change*. Birmingham, West Midlands Partnerships for Mental Health.

Bailey, D. (Ed.) (2000) *At the Core of Mental Health*. Brighton, Pavilion.

Bainbridge, M. (2002) 'Carers are People Too', *Mental Health Today*. June 2002.

Bamber, C. (2001) 'Modernising Crisis Services: What Do Users want from 24-hour Services?' *The Mental Health Review*. 6: 1, March, 2001.

Bamford, T. (1982) *Managing Social Work*. London, Tavistock/Methuen.

Bamford, T. (2000) *Integrated Health and Social Care in Northern Ireland: Myth and Reality*. Paper for A.D.S.S. Seminar, August 2000.

Banks, S. (1995) *Ethics and Values in Social Work*. London, Macmillan.

Banyard, R., Jones, H. T., Hampshaw, S. and Dunn, A. (2002) 'Social Skills', *Health Service Journal*. 29th Aug.

Barnes, D. and Brandon, T. with Webb, T. (2000) *Independent Specialist Advocacy in England and Wales: Recommendations for Good Practice*. University of Durham Centre for Applied Social Studies.

Bates, P. (Ed.) (2002) *Working for Inclusion: Making Social Inclusion a Reality for People with Severe Mental Health Problems*. London, Sainsbury Centre for Mental Health.

Behan, D. and Loft, L. (1999) 'Primary Care Groups: A Social Services Perspective', *Managing Community Care*. 7: 2, Apr.

Benedict of Nursia (circa. 540 A.D.) Translation Fry T. (Ed.) (1982) *The Rule of St. Benedict*. Minnesota, The Liturgical Press.

Beresford, P. (2002) 'Making User Involvement', *Professional Social Work*. June, 2002.

Beresford, P. (2002) 'Encouraging Caring Communities', *Mental Health Today*. February, 2002.

Biestek, F. (1976) *The Casework Relationship*, London, George Allen and Unwin (originally published in 1957 by the Loyola University Press).

Braye, S. and Preston-Shoot, M. (1995) *Empowering Practice in Social Care*. Buckingham, Open University Press.

Brayne, H. and Martin, G. (1999) 6th edn. *Law for Social Workers*. London, Blackstone.

Brechin, A., Brown, H. and Eby, M. (Eds.) (2000) *Critical Practice in Health and Social Care*. London, Sage/Open University Press.

Brewin, M. (1996) *Respectful Privacy, Dignity and Religious and Cultural Beliefs: The Needs of Patients from Different Ethnic Backgrounds*. Bath Health Promotion Unit/Wiltshire Health Authority.

British Association of Social Workers (1975, amended 1986) *A Code of Ethics for Social Work*, BASW.

British Association of Social Workers (2002) *Response to the Consultation on the Draft Mental Health Bill*, BASW.

British Association of Social Workers (2002) *The Code of Ethics for Social Workers*, BASW.

Bucknall, B. (1981) *Ursula K. Le Guin*, New York, Frederick Ungar.

Burke, R. and Cooper, C. (Eds. 2000) *The Organisation in Crisis: Downsizing, Restructuring and Privatisation*, Oxford. Blackwell Publishers.

Butler, A. and Pritchard, C. (1983) *Social Work and Mental Illness*, London, Macmillan.

Butrym, Z. (1976) *The Nature of Social Work*, London, Macmillan.

C.C.E.T.S.W. (2000) *Guidance on the Implementation of Assuring Quality for Mental Health Social Work*, London C.C.E.T.S.W., April 2000.

Campbell, J. and McLaughlin, J. (2000) 'The Joined Up Management of Adult Health and Social Care Services in Northern Ireland', *Managing Community Care*, Vol. 8, No. 5.

Cassam, E. and Gupta, H. (1992) *Quality Assurance for Social Care Agencies*, Harlow, Longman.

Challis, D., Chessum, R., Chesterman, J., Luckett, R. and Traske, K. (1990) *Case Management in Social and Health Care*, Canterbury, University of Kent Personal Social Services Research Unit.

Chantler, K. (2002) 'The Invisibility of Black Women in Mental Health Services', *The Mental Health Review*, Vol. 7, Issue 1, March 2002.

Clark, C. and Lapsley, I. (Eds.) (1996) *Planning and Costing Community Care*, Edinburgh, Jessica Kingsley Press.

Clarke, J. (Ed.) (1993) *A Crisis in Care?: Challenges to Social Work*, Buckingham, Open University/SAGE.

Clayton, M. (2002) 'Valued Beyond Doubt', *Community Care*, 23rd–29th May, 2002.

Coleman, R. (1998) *The Politics of the Madhouse*, Handsell Publishing.

Collins, J. (2001) *Good to Great*, London, Random House Business.

Collins, J. and Porras, J. (2000, 3rd edition) *Built to Last: Successful Habits of Visionary Companies*, London, Random House Business .

Cooper, A. (2002) 'Keeping our Heads: Preserving Therapeutic Values in a Time of Change', *Journal of Social Work Practice*, Vol. 6: No. 1, March 2002.

Cooper, C. L. and Makin, P. (1984, second revised edition) *Psychology for Managers*, Trowbridge, The British Psychological Society and Macmillan.

Cope, R. (1989) 'The Compulsory Detention of Afro-Caribbeans under the Mental Health Act', *New Community*, 15 (3): 343–56.

Copsey, N. (1997) *Keeping Faith: The Provision of Community Health Services Within a Multi-Faith Context*, The Sainsbury Centre for Mental Health.

Copsey, N. (2001) *Forward in Faith: An Experiment in Building Bridges Between Ethnic Communities and Mental Health Services in East London*, Sainsbury Centre for Mental Health.

Cormack, D. (1988), *Team Spirit*, MARC.

Coulshead, V. (1988) *Social Work Practice: An Introduction*, London, Macmillan.

Coulshead, V. and Orme, J. (1998, 3rd edition) *Social Work Practice*, London, Macmillan.

Davies, M. (1981 1st edition) *The Essential Social Worker*, London: Heinemann Educational/Community Care.

Davies, M. (1994, 3rd edition) *The Essential Social Worker*, Aldershot, Gower.

Dear, M. and Wolch, J. (1987) *Landscapes of Despair: From Deinstitutionalisation to Homelessness*, Oxford, Polity Press.

Department of Health (2002) *Local Health Policy Implementation Guide: Community Mental Health Teams*, London, Department of Health, June 2002.

Department of Health (2002) *Mental Health Policy Implementation Guide: Adult Acute Inpatient Care Provision*, London, HMSO, April 2002.

Department of Health, (2001) *The Road to Recovery: The Government's Vision for Mental Health Care*, London, HMSO, November 2001.

Desai, S. and Bevan, D. (1998) 'Anti-Racist Practice: The Role of the Social Worker in Managing Different Perspectives in Care: *The Journal of Practice and Development*, Vol. 7, 1998.

Desai, S. and Bevan, D. (2002) 'Race and Culture' in Thompson, N. (Ed.) (2002) *Loss and Grief: A Guide for Human Services Practitioners*, London, Palgrave.

DHSS (1975) *Better Services for the Mentally Ill*, CMND 6233, London, HMSO.

Dickens, P. and Gilbert, P. (1979) *The State and the Housing Question*, University of Sussex Monograph, July 1979.

Double, D. (2002) 'Redressing The Imbalance', *Mental Health Today*, September, 2002.

Duggan, M. (2002) 'What is the Knowledge Base and Where Does it Come From?': *Thoughts from the Social Perspectives Network Study Day*, SPN, 1st May 2002.

Duggan, M. with Cooper, A. and Foster, J. (2002) *Modernising the Social Model in Mental Health: A Discussion Paper*, Social Perspectives Network, January 2002.

Egan, G. (1975) *The Skilled Helper*, California, Brooks/Cole.

Egan, G. (2002, 7th edition) *The Skilled Helper*, California, Brooks/Cole.

England, H. (1986) *Social Work as Art: Making Sense for Good Practice*, London, Allen and Unwin.

Faulkner, A. and Bassett, T. (2002) 'Bringing the Framework to Life', *Mental Health Today*, March 2002.

Fernando, S. (Ed.) (1995) *Mental Health in a Multi-Ethnic Society: A Multi-Disciplinary Handbook*, London, Routledge.

Firth, M. T. (1999), 'Conversing with Clients: A Generic Approach to Mental Health Needs Assessment', *Practice*, Vol. 11, No. 2, 1999.

Firth, M. T. (2000) *MANCAS Guide and Schedule*, Central Manchester Health Care NHS. Trust.

Flamholtz, E. and Randle, Y. (1989) *The Inner Game of Management*, London, Hutchinson.

George, M. (2002) 'Take Your Partners', *Mental Health Today*, April, 2002.

Gilbert, P. (1985) *Mental Handicap: A Practical Guide for Social Workers*, London, Business Press International.

Gilbert, P. (1992) *Cultural Change in a Public Welfare Agency – Antecedents, Process and Consequences*, Unpublished MBA Thesis, Roffey Park Institute/Sussex University.

Gilbert, P. (2003/4, forthcoming) *Managing Change in Organisations*, Wrexham, Learning Curve Publishing.

Gilbert, P. and Scragg, T. (1992) *Managing to Care*, Sutton, Reed Business Publishing.

Gilbert, P. and Spooner, B. (1982), 'Strength in Unity', *Community Care*, 28th October 1982.

Gilbert, P. and Thompson, N. (2002) *Supervision and Leadership Skills: A Training Resource*, Wrexham, Learning Curve Publishing.

Glover, H. and Allott, P. (2002) *Developing a Recovery Platform for Mental Health Service Delivery for People with Mental Illness/Distress in England*, First Draft Executive Summary, NIMHE Connections Conference, Newcastle-upon-Tyne, June 2002.

Goffman, E. (1970) *Stigma: Notes on the Management of Spoiled Identity*, Harmondsworth, Penguin.

Goleman, D. (1998) 'What Makes a Leader?', *Harvard Business Review*, Nov–Dec 1998.

Goleman, D. (1996) *Emotional Intelligence*, London, Bloomsbury.

Griffiths, R. (1988) *Community Care: Agenda For Action*, London, HMSO.

Gulliver, P., Peck, E. and Towell, D. (2000) 'Evaluation of the Implementation of the Mental Health Review in Somerset: Methodology', *Managing Community Care*, Vol. 8, No. 3, June 2000.

Gulliver, P., Peck, E. and Towell, D. (2000) 'Evaluation of the Implementation of the Mental Health Review in Somerset: Baseline Data', *Managing Community Care*, Vol. 8, No. 4, August 2000.

Gulliver, P., Peck, E. and Towell, D. (2001) 'Evaluation of the Implementation of the Mental Health Review in Somerset: Results After Fifteen Months of Data Collection', *Managing Community Care*, Vol. 9, No. 1.

Gulliver, P., Peck, E. and Towell, D. (2002) *Modernising Partnerships: Evaluation of the Implementation of the Mental Health Review in Somerset: Final Report*, Institute for Applied Health and Social Policy, Kings College, London.

Gulliver, P., Peck, E. and Towell, D. (2002) 'Evaluation of the Integration of Health and Social Services in Somerset: Part 2 – Lessons for Other Localities, *M.C.C., Vol 10, issue 3, June 2002.*

Hampden-Turner, C. (1990) *Corporate Culture: From Vicious to Virtuous Circles*, London, Hutchinson Business.

Handy, C. (1979) *Gods of Management*, London, Pan.

Handy, C. (1985 3rd edition) *Understanding Organisations*, London, Penguin Books.

Hanvey, C. and Philpot, T. (1994) *Practising Social Work*, London, Routledge.

Harding, T. and Beresford, P. (1996), *The Standards We Expect: What Service Users Want from Social Services Workers*, London: National Institute for Social Work.

Harrison, R. and Stokes, H. (1990) *Diagnosing Organisational Culture*, Sussex, Roffey Park Management Institute.

Hart, L. (1997) *Phone at Nine Just to Say You're Alive*, London, Pan Books.

Harvey, D. (1990) *The Condition of Postmodernity: An Enquiry into the Origin of Cultural Change*, Oxford, Blackwell.

Harvey-Jones, J. (1986) *Making it Happen: Reflections on Leadership*, Glasgow, William Collins.

Health Education Authority, *Promoting Mental Health: The Role of Faith Communities – Jewish and Christian Perspectives*, London, HEA.

Heimler, E. (1967) *Mental Illness and Social Work*, Middlesex, Penguin.

Heller, T., Reynolds, J., Gomm, R., Muston, R., Patison, S. (Eds.) (1996) *Mental Health Matters: A Reader*, London Open University Press.

Hetherington, R., Baistow, K., Catz, I., Mesie, J., Trowell, J. (2001) *The Welfare of Children with Mentally Ill Parents: Learning from Inter-country Comparisons*, Chichester, John Wiley.

Hewitt, P. (2001) *So You Think You're Mad: Seven Practical Steps to Mental Health*, Handsell Publishing.

Hill, C. (1972) *The World Turned Upside Down: Radical Ideas During the English Revolution*, London, Temple Smith.

Hoffman, E. (1989) *Lost in Translation: A Life in a New Language*, London, Heinemann.

Hofstede, G. (1980) *Cultures Consequences*, Beverley Hills, SAGE.

Hoggett, B. (1984, 2nd edition) *Mental Health Law*, London, Sweet and Maxwell.

House of Commons Social Services Committee (1985) Second Report of the House of Commons Social Services Committee: *Community Care*, London, HMSO.

Hudson, B. (2002) 'Ten Reasons Not to Trust Care Trusts', *M.C.C.*, Vol. 10, Issue 2, April 2002.

Hughes, L. (2001) 'New Culture, New Territory, New Professions?', in Allen, I. (Ed.) (2001) *Social Care and Health: A New Deal?* London, Policy Studies Institute/University of Westminster.

Jamison, K. R. (1997) *An Unquiet Mind: A Memoir of Moods and Madness*, London, Macmillan/Picador.

Jenkins, S. (1995) *Accountable to None: The Tory Nationalisation of Britain*, London, Hamish Hamilton.

Jenkins, R., McCulloch, A., Friedli, L., Parker, C. (2002) *Developing a National Mental Health Policy*, Hove, Psychology Press/Maudsley Monographs.

Johnson, G. and Scholes, K. (1989 3rd edition) *Exploring Corporate Strategy: Text and Cases*, Hemel Hempstead, Prentice Hall.

Jones, K. (1972) *A History of the Mental Health Services*, London, Routledge and Kegan Paul.

Jones, K. (1988) *Experience in Mental Health: Community Care and Social Policy*, London, SAGE.

Jones, R. (2001, 7th edition) *Mental Health Act Manual*, London, Sweet and Maxwell.

Jordan, B. (1976) *Freedom and the Welfare State*, London, Routledge and Kegan Paul.

Jordan, B. (1984) *Invitation to Social Work*, Oxford, Martin Robertson.

Kardong, T. (1988) *The Benedictines*, Dublin, Dominican Publications.

Kelley, R. (1988) 'In Praise of Followers', *Havard Business Review*, November – December 1988.

Kermode, F. (Ed.) (1975) *Selected Prose of T. S. Eliot*, London, Faber.

Kerr, S. (1983) *Making Ends Meet*, London: Bedford Square Press.

Kohen, D. (Ed.) (2000) *Women and Mental Health*, London, Routledge.

Kotter, J. P. (1995) 'Leading Change: Why Transformation Efforts Fail', *Harvard Business Review*, March/April, 1995.

Kotter, J. P. (1996) *Leading Change*, Boston, Harvard Business School Press.

Kouzes, J. and Posner, B. (1990) 'The Credibility Factor: What Followers Expect from their Leaders', *Management Review*, January 1990.

Kuhn, T. (1962) *The Structure of Scientific Revolutions*, Chicago, Chicago University Press.

Le Guin, U. K. (1971) *The Lathe of Heaven*, London, Victor Gollancz.

Le Guin, U. K. (1973) *The Farthest Shore*, London, Victor Vollancz.

Le Guin, U. K. (1984) 'S.Q.', *In the Compass Rose*, London, Panther.

Le Guin, U. K. (1974) *The Dispossessed*, London, Victor Gollancz.

Le Mesurier, N. and Cumella, S. (2001) 'The Rough Road and the Smooth Road', *Managing Community Care*, Vol. 9, No. 1.

Leeds Mental Health Unit, (1997) '*A Little More Time, Too*': A Consumer Survey of the Leeds Mental Health Social Work Services, Leeds Social Services, January 1997.

Leggatt, A. (March 2001) *Tribunals for Users: One System, One Service*, London: The Stationery Office, March 2001.

Lewis, J. and Glennerster, H. (1996) *Implementing the New Community Care*, Buckingham, Open University Press.

Macdonald, G. and Sheldon, B. (1997) Community Care Services for the Mentally Ill: Consumers Views. *International Journal of Social Psychiatry*. 43: 1, 35–55.

Mackay, R. et al. (2001) *Report of the Independent Enquiry into the Care and Treatment Afforded to Benjamin Rathbone*, Leicestershire Health Authority, November 2001.

Magee, B. (1973) *Popper*, London, Fontana.

Maslow, A. H. (1965) *Eupsychiam Management*, Homewood, Illinois, Irwin-Dorsey.

Means, R. and Smith, R. (1994) *Community Care Policy and Practice*, London, Macmillan.

Mental Health Act Commission (2001) *The Mental Health Act Commission 9th Biennial Report 1999–2001*, London, HMSO.

Mental Health Foundation, (2002) *Taken Seriously: The Somerset Spirituality Project*, London, Mental Health Foundation.

Mental Health Foundation, (2000) *Strategies for Living*, London, Mental Health Foundation.

Mental Health Foundation (1999) *The Fundamental Facts*, London, Mental Health Foundation.

Mental Health Foundation, (1997) *Knowing Our Own Minds: A Survey of How People in Emotional Distress Take Control of Their Lives*, Mental Health Foundation.

Midwinter, E. (1994) *The Development of Social Welfare in Britain*, Buckingham, Open University Press.

Morrell, M. and Capparell, S. (2001) *Shackleton's Way: Leadership Lessons from the Great Antarctic Explorer*, London, Nicholas Brealey.

Morris, D. (2001) 'Citizenship and Community in Mental Health: A Joint National Programme for Social Inclusion and Community Partnership', *The Mental Health Review*, Vol. 6, Issue 3, September 2001.

Murray, A., Shepherd, G., Onyett, S., Muijen, M. (1997) *More Than a Friend: The Role of Support*

Workers in Community Mental Health Services, London, Sainsbury Centre for Mental Health.

National Institute for Mental Health in England, (2001) *The National Institute for Mental Health in England: Role and Function*, London HMSO, June 2001.

National Institute for Mental Health in England, (2002) *First Year Strategy for NIMHE: Meeting the Implementation Challenge in Mental Health*, Department of Health, June 2002.

Newman, J. (1996) *Shaping Organisational Cultures in Local Government*, London, Pitman.

Neyroud, P. and Beckley, A. (2001) *Policing, Ethics and Human Rights*, Devon, Willan.

Nocon, A. and Qureshi, H. (1996) *Outcomes of Community Care for Users and Carers*, Buckingham, Open University Press.

NSF, *Meeting the Spiritual Needs of People with a Severe Mental Illness*, Policy Statement No. 40.

Oldham Social Services and Oldham NHS Trust (2002) *Mental Health Social Work in Oldham*, Oldham Social Services/Oldham NHS Trust, January 2002.

Olsen, M. R. (Ed.) (1984) *Social Work and Mental Health*, London, Tavistock.

O'Neill, G. (1997) *In the Context of a Multi-Disciplinary Duty System, Are There Differences in the Practice and Division of Labour Between Community Psychiatric Nurses and Mental Health Social Workers?*, Unpublished MA Thesis, University of Lancaster, March 1997.

Onyett, S., Pillinger, T. and Muijen, M. (1995) *Making Community Mental Health Teams Work*, London, Sainsbury Centre for Mental Health.

Padgett, N. and Swannell, G. (1997) *Diamonds Behind My Eyes*, London, Victor Gollancz.

Parton, N. and O'Byrne, P. (2000) *Constructive Social Work: Towards a New Practice*, London, Macmillan.

Payne, C. (1988) 'When Management Skills are Part of Basic Practice', *Social Work Today*, 23rd June 1988.

Payne, M. (1982), *Working in Teams*, London, Macmillan.

Payne, M. (2002) 'Balancing The Equation', *Professional Social Work*, January 2002.

Peck, E., Gulliver, P., Towell, D. (2002) *Modernising Partnerships: An Evaluation of Somerset's Innovations in the Commissioning and Organisation of Mental Health Services, Final Report*, London, Institute for Applied Health and Social Policy, March 2002.

Pendegarth, Y. (2002) *Woman Speak Out: Women's Experiences of Using Mental Health Services and Proposals for Change*, Resisters, Leeds Women's and Mental Health Action Group.

Peters, T. and Austin, N. (1986) *A Passion for Excellence: The Leadership Difference*, Glasgow, William Collins/Fontana Paperbacks.

Perkins, R. (2002) 'Are you (really) Being Served?', *Mental Health Today*, September, 2002.

Phillips, C., Palfrey, C. and Thomas, P. (1994) *Evaluating Health and Social Care*, London, Macmillan.

Philpot, T. (Ed.) (1986) *Social Work: A Christian Perspective*, Tring, Lion Publishing.

Pierson, J. (2002) *Tackling Social Exclusion*, Sutton, Community Care.

Porter, R. (2002) *Madness: A Brief History*, Oxford, Oxford University Press.

Preston-Shoot, M. (1996) 'Wither Social Work? Social Work, Social Policy and Law at an Interface: Confronting the Challenges and Realising the Potential in Work with People Needing Care or Services' *The Liverpool Law Review*, XVIII.

Proehl, R. A. (2001) *Organisational Change in the Human Services*, Thousand Oaks, California, SAGE.

Ramon, S. (2001) *Options and Dilemmas Facing British Mental Health Social Work*, Paper for the Conference on Reducing the Biomedical Dominance of Psychiatry, 27th April 2001.

Ramsay, R., Gerada, C., Mars, S., Szmukler, G. (Eds.) (2001) *Mental Illness: A Handbook for Carers*, London, Jessica Kingsley.

Reed, M. (2002) 'The Practitioner's Perspective', *Professional Social Work*, April 2002.

Ritchie, J. H., Dick and Lingham, R. (1994) *The Report of the Enquiry into the Care and Treatment of Christopher Clunis*, London, H.M.S.O.

Rogers, C. (1961) *Client-centred Therapy: It's Current Practice, Theory and Implications*, London, Constable.

Rolheiser, R. (1998) *Seeking Spirituality*, London, Hodder and Stoughton.

Rose, D. (2001) Users' Voices: *The Perspectives of Mental Health Service Users on Community and Hospital Care*, London, The Sainsbury Centre for Mental Health.

Rushton, A. and Davies, P. (1984) *Social Work and Health Care*, London, Heinemann Educational.

Russell, A., Haldane, J., Russell, T. (2001 4th edition) 'Positive Practice in Mental Health', *Breakthrough*, July 2001.

SSI (2001) *Inspection of Mental Health Services*, London Borough of Hounslow, London, HMSO, June 2001.

SSI (2001) *Inspection of Mental Health Services*, Southend-on-Sea Borough Council, London, HMSO, September 2001.

Sainsbury Centre for Mental Health,(1998) *Acute Problems: A Survey of the Quality of Care in Acute Psychiatric Wards: Briefing Paper 4*, London, SCMH, November 1998.

Sainsbury Centre for Mental Health, (2000) *An Executive Briefing on the Implications of the Human Rights Act 1998 for Mental Health Services: Briefing Paper 12*, London, SCMH, December 2000.

Sainsbury Centre for Mental Health, (2000) *On Your Doorstep: Community Organisations and Mental Health*, London, SCMH.

Sainsbury Centre for Mental Health, (2000) *Taking Your Partners: Using Opportunities for Inter-Agency Partnership in Mental Health*, London, SCMH.

Sainsbury Centre for Mental Health, (2001) *An Executive Briefing on White Paper Reforming the Mental Health Act: Briefing Paper 14*, London, SCMH, March 2001.

Sainsbury Centre for Mental Health, (2002) *An Executive Briefing on 'Working for Inclusion': Briefing Paper 15*, London, SCMH.

Sainsbury Centre for Mental Health, (2002) *Breaking The Circles of Fear: A Review of the Relationship Between Mental Health Services and African and Caribbean Communities*, London, SCMH.

Schein, E. (1985) *Organisational Culture and Leadership*, San Francisco, Jossey-Bass Press.

Scott, M. C. (2000) *Re-inspiring the Corporation*, Chichester, John Wiley.

Scull, A. (1984, 2nd edition) *Decarceration: Community Treatment and the Deviant – A Radical View*, Cambridge, Polity Press.

Shaw, I. and Gould, N. (2001) *Qualitative Research in Social Work*, London, SAGE.

Shaw, I. and Middleton, H. (2001) 'Recognising Depression in Primary Care', *Primary Care Mental Health*, Vol. 5, No. 2.

Shaw, P. (2002) *Changing Conversations in Organisations*, London, Routledge.

Sheppard, M. (1995) *Care Management and the New Social Work: A Critical Analaysis*, London, Whiting and Birch.

Slay, G. (2002) 'A Question of Judgement', *Professional Social Work*, July 2002.

Smale, G., Tuson, G., Ahmad, B., Darvill, G., Domoney, L., Sainsbury, E. (1994) *Negotiating Care in the Commmunity*, London, HMSO.

Smale, G., Tuson, G. and Statham, D. (2000) *Social Work and Social Problems: Working*

Towards Social Inclusion and Social Change, London, Palgrave.

Spicker, P. (1995) *Social Policy: Themes and Approaches*, Hemel Hempstead, Prentice Hall.

Stanley, N. and Manthorpe, J. (2001) 'Reading Mental Health Enquiries: Messages for Social Work', *Journal of Social Work*, vol. 1, No. 1.

Stevenson, O. (1971) 'Knowledge for Social Work', *British Journal of Social Work*, Vol. 1, No. 2, Summer 1971.

Swinton, J. (2001) *Spirituality and Mental Health Care: Rediscovering a 'Forgotten' Dimension*, London, Jessica Kingsley.

Taylor, C. and White, S. (2000) *Practising Reflexivity in Health and Welfare*, Buckingham, Open University Press.

Tew, J. (2002) 'Going Social: Championing an Holistic Model of Mental Distress Within Professional Education', *Social Work Education*, Vol. 1, No. 2, April 2002.

Thompson, N. (1992) *Existentialism and Social Work*, Aldershot, Avebury.

Thompson, N. (1998) *Promoting Equality*, London, Macmillan.

Thompson, N. (2000) *Understanding Social Work: Preparing for Practice*, London, Macmillan.

Thompson, N. (2001) 'Working Together Across Disciplines', *N. T. Research*, Vol. 6, No. 5, 2001.

Timms, N. and R. (1977) *Perspectives in Social Work*, London, Routledge and Kegan Paul.

Titmuss, R. M. (1961) Paper by Professor Richard Titmuss at the Annual Conference of the National Association for Mental Health, 1961, reproduced in Titmuss, R. M. (1968) *Commitment to Welfare*, London, Allen and Unwin.

Topor, A. (2000) *Chronic Illness(es) and Recovery*, Unpublished Paper, November 2000.

Ulas, M. and Connor, A. (Eds.) (1999) *Mental Health and Social Work*, London, Jessica Kingsley.

Utting, W. (2002) 'Preaching What we Practise', *Professional Social Work*, June 2002.

Wallace Hadrill, J. M. (1971) *Early Germanic Kingship in England and on the Continent*, London, Oxford University Press.

Weaver, (1998) Case Management Conference in Oklahoma quoted in Allott, P. and Loganathan, L. (2002) *Discovering Hope for Recovery from a British Perspective: A review of a Sample of Recovery Literature, Implications for Practice and Systems Change*.

Webster, A. (2001) 'Embodied Leadership', *Ministry*, Summer 2001.

Westwood, S., Couloute, J., Desai, S., Matthew, P. and Piper, A. (1989) *Sadness In My Heart:*

Racism and Mental Health, Leicester Black Mental Health Group, Leicester University.

Williams, J., and Scott, S. (2002) 'Service Responses to Women with Mental Health Needs', *The Mental Health Review*, Vol. 7, Issue 1, March 2002.

Williams, R. (2000) *Lost Icons: Reflections on Cultural Bereavement*, Edinburgh, Continuum Books.

Winnicott, D. (1963 essay, published 1965) 'The Mentally Ill on Your Caseload', *The Maturational Processes of the Facilitating Environment*, London, Hogarth Press (reprinted Karnac Books, 1990).

Winterson, J. (2000) *The Power Book*, London, Jonathan Cape Ltd.

Woodward, A. and Kohli, M. (2001) *Inclusions and Exclusions in European Societies*, London, Routledge.

Younghusband, E, Younghusband Report, 1959, *Report of the Working Party on Social Workers in the Local Authority Health and Welfare Services*, London, HMSO.

Younghusband, E. (1978) *Social Work in Britain: 1950–1975*, London, Unwin.

Zohar, D. and Marshall, I. (2000) *S.Q: Spiritual Intelligence, The Ultimate Intelligence*, London, Bloomsbury.